HBJ HEALTH
Revised Edition

Orange

Consulting Health Educators

Carolyn C. Burton
Formerly Coordinator of Student Teaching in Health and Physical Education
The University of Texas at Austin

David Poehler, Ph.D.
Assistant Professor
Department of Health Education
University of Alabama
Birmingham, Alabama

Romaine B. Sullivan, M.P.H.
Teacher and Department Chairperson
Thomas Aquinas High School
San Marcos, California

William D. Utter, Ed.D.
Formerly Director of Health and Drug Education
Alamance County Schools
North Carolina

Consulting Health Specialists

Judy Chapin
Renal Dietitian
Mt. Zion Hospital and Medical Center
San Francisco

Martin Heinstein, Ph.D.
Professor of Psychology
San Francisco State University

Edward Kormondy, Ph.D.
Provost and Professor of Biology
University of Southern Maine

Allison Nicholas Metz, M.D.
Fellow, American Academy of Dermatology
Clinical Instructor
Department of Dermatology
University of California, San Francisco

Lance E. Percy, Ed. D.
Licensed Mental Health Counselor
New Smyrna Beach, Florida

Irene Savostin-Asling, D.D.S., Ph.D.

Ronald T. Stafford, M.D.
Presbyterian Hospital
San Francisco

Ronald R. Sunde, D.D.S.

Scarlette M. Wilson, B.S. in Pharmacy; M.D.
Assistant Clinical Professor of Ophthalmology
University of California, San Francisco
Chief of Ophthalmology
Ralph K. Davies Medical Center
San Francisco

HBJ HARCOURT BRACE JOVANOVICH, PUBLISHERS
Orlando   San Diego   Chicago   Dallas

PHOTOGRAPH ACKNOWLEDGMENTS
COVER: HBJ Photo/Frank Wing
Key: t(top), b(bottom), c(center), l(left), r(right)
Page 3, HBJ Photo/Josephine Coatsworth; 4, HBJ Photo/Josephine Coatsworth; 5, HBJ Photo/Norman Prince; 6, HBJ Photo/Norman Prince; 7, HBJ Photo/Josephine Coatsworth; 8, HBJ Photo/Josephine Coatsworth; 9(l), HBJ Photo/Josephine Coatsworth; 9(r), HBJ Photo/Norman Prince; 10, HBJ Photo/Norman Prince; 12(l), HBJ Photo/Josephine Coatsworth; 12(r), HBJ Photo; 13, HBJ Photo/Josephine Coatsworth; 14, HBJ Photo/Elliott Varner Smith; 15, HBJ Photo/Marcy Maloy; 16(r), HBJ Photo/Marcy Maloy; 17, Norman Prince; 18(l), Lorraine Rorke; 18(r), American Women's Himalayan Expedition; 19, HBJ Photo/Josephine Coatsworth; 20, HBJ Photo/Norman Prince; 22, HBJ Photo/Josephine Coatsworth; 24, HBJ Photo/Norman Prince; 27, R. Rowan; 28(l), Carolina Biological Supply Co.; 28(c,r), Martin M. Rotker/Taurus Photos; 29(t), Paul Fusco/Magnum Photos; 29(l), Phil Degginger/Bruce Coleman, Inc.; 29(c), Alfred Owczarzak/Taurus Photos; 29(r), Stepanowiez/Bruce Coleman, Inc.; 29(rc), HBJ Photo; 30, HBJ Photo/Frank Wing; 32, HBJ Photo; 35, Elliott Varner Smith; 38, HBJ Photo/Norman Prince; 41. R. Rowan; 44, Carolina Biological Supply Co.; 49, Bill O'Connor/Peter Arnold, Inc.; 52, Jerry Wachter/F.O.S., Inc.; 54, Sensory Aids Corp.; 58, HBJ Photo/Norman Prince; 64, HBJ Photo/Erik Arnesen; 65, HBJ Photo/Erik Arnesen; 66(l) Courtesy of the Summerfield Family; 66 (r), HBJ Photo/Josephine Coatsworth; 67(t), HBJ Photo/Josephine Coatsworth; 67(b), HBJ Photo/Josephine Coatsworth; 69(r), Synapse Productions; 70, HBJ Photo/Elliott Varner Smith; 71, Don Kelly; 73, Leonard Freed/Magnum Photos; 74, HBJ Photo/Norman Prince; 75, HBJ Photo/Elliott Varner Smith; 76, HBJ Photo/Frank Wing; 77, HBJ Photo/Frank Wing; 79, HBJ Photo/Elliott Varner Smith; 84, HBJ Photo/Elliott Varner Smith; 85, HBJ Photo/Elliott Varner Smith; 86, HBJ Photo/Norman Prince; 88, HBJ Photo/Bob Powals; 91(both), American Dental Association, Reprinted by Permission; 93, Sherry L. Bryan; 94, Manfred Kage/Peter Arnold, Inc.; 96(l), HBJ Photo; 96 (r), HBJ Photo/Norman Prince; 97, HBJ Photo/Elliott Varner Smith; 98, HBJ Photo/Josephine Coatsworth; 99, HBJ Photo/Norman Prince; 100, HBJ Photo/Elliott Varner Smith; 106, Joyce R. Wilson; 107, Joyce R. Wilson; 108, HBJ Photo/Elliott Varner Smith; 109, HBJ Photo/Norman Prince; 111(l), HBJ Photo/Elliott Varner Smith; 111 (r), HBJ Photo/Norman Prince; 112, HBJ Photo/Norman Prince; 113, Pat Fukahara; 114, HBJ Photo/Norman Prince; 115, HBJ Photo/Norman Prince; 116, HBJ Photo/Norman Prince; 117, HBJ Photo/Norman Prince; 118(l), HBJ Photo/Norman Prince; 118(r), Paul Fusco/Magnum Photos; 119, HBJ Photo/Norman Prince; 120, HBJ Photo/Norman Prince; 121, HBJ Photo/Elliott Varner Smith; 122, HBJ Photo/Norman Prince; 123, HBJ Photo/Elliott Varner Smith; 124, HBJ Photo/Norman Prince; 127, HBJ Photo/Elliott Varner Smith; 133, Carolina Biological Supply Co.; 134, HBJ Photo/Elliott Varner Smith; 135, HBJ Photo/Elliott Varner Smith; 136(l,c), Manfred Kage/Peter Arnold, Inc.; 136(r), Carolina Biological Supply Co.; 137(t), Courtesy Dr. Robley C. Williams, Virus Laboratory, University of California, Berkeley; 137(c), Stanford University; 137(b), Carolina Biological Supply Co.; 139, Lennart Nilsson/BEHOLD MAN, Little, Brown and Co., Boston; 141, HBJ Photo; 142, HBJ Photo/Norman Prince; 143, HBJ Photo/Norman Prince; 144(l), Runk/Schoen-berger/Grant Heilman Photography; 144(r), HBJ Photo/Norman Prince; 145, HBJ Photo/Norman Prince; 146, HBJ Photo/Norman Prince; 147, Runk/Schoenberger/Grant Heilman Photography; 148, Runk/Schoenberger/Grant Heilman Photography; 149, HBJ Photo/Norman Prince; 150, Lennart Nilsson/BEHOLD MAN, Little, Brown and Co., Boston; 152, Ken Regan/Camera 5; 153, Guy Gillette; 160, HBJ Photo/Norman Prince; 161, HBJ Photo/Norman Prince; 162, HBJ Photo/Norman Prince; 163, HBJ Photo/Norman Prince; 164, HBJ Photo/Norman Prince; 165, HBJ Photo/Norman Prince; 166(t), HBJ Photo/Elliott Varner Smith; 166(b), HBJ Photo/Norman Prince; 167 (l), HBJ Photo/Norman Prince; 167(r), HBJ Photo/Elliott Varner Smith; 168, Synapse Productions; 169, HBJ Photo/Norman Prince; 171, HBJ Photo/Elliott Varner Smith; 172, HBJ Photo/Norman Prince; 174, American Cancer Society; 176, Syd Greenberg/Photo Researchers, Inc.; 178, HBJ Photo; 179, Alec Duncan 1982; 181, HBJ Photo/Elliott Varner Smith; 182, HBJ Photo/Norman Prince; 183, HBJ Photo/Elliott Varner Smith; 188, Trudi Beth Edelman; 189, Trudi Beth Edelman; 190, HBJ Photo/Norman Prince; 191, HBJ Photo/Elliott Varner Smith; 193, HBJ Photo/Norman Prince; 194, Star-News Newspapers; 195, HBJ Photo/Norman Prince; 196, HBJ Photo/Norman Prince; 197, HBJ Photo/Elliott Varner Smith; 198, HBJ Photo; 199, HBJ Photo/Norman Prince; 200, HBJ Photo/Norman Prince; 201, HBJ Photo/Erik Arnesen; 202, HBJ Photo/Norman Prince; 203, HBJ Photo; 204, HBJ Photo/Norman Prince; 205, HBJ Photo/Elliott Varner Smith; 207, Red Cross; 208, D.F. Anthony; 209, HBJ Photo/Norman Prince; 210, HBJ Photo/Norman Prince; 211(l), Owen Kahn; 211(r), HBJ Photo/Elliott Varner Smith; 212, HBJ Photo/Elliott Varner Smith; 213, HBJ Photo/Elliott Varner Smith; 215, HBJ Photo/Norman Prince; 218, Tom Tracy; 219, Tom Tracy; 220, Sonia Katchian/Black Star; 221, HBJ Photo/Elliott Varner Smith; 222 (l), HBJ Photo; 222(r), HBJ Photo/Elliott Varner Smith; 223(l), Jan Halaska/Photo Researchers, Inc. 1980; 223(r), HBJ Photo/Frank Wing; 224, HBJ Photo/Erik Arnesen; 225, HBJ Photo/Frank Wing; 226 (l), HBJ Photo/Susan Lohwasser; 226(r), HBJ Photo/Erik Arnesen; 227 (t), HBJ Photo/Norman Prince; 227(b), Tom Tracy; 228, HBJ Photo/Norman Prince; 229, HBJ Photo/Norman Prince; 230, HBJ Photo/Elliott Varner Smith; 231(l), Grant Heilman Photography; 231 (r), Karen R. Preuss; 232(l), Environmental Protection Agency; 232 (r), HBJ Photo/Phil Toy; 233, The Bunker Hill Co.; 234, Tom Tracy; 235, Tom Tracy; 236, Tom Tracy; 237, Phil Toy; 238, HBJ Photo/Norman Prince; 239(l), Runk/Schoenberger/Grant Heilman Photography; 239 (r). Charles Harbutt; 240, Don Carstens; 241(l), Tom Tracy; 241 (r), HBJ Photo/Dan DeWilde; 242, HBJ Photo/Erik Arnesen.

ART ACKNOWLEDGMENTS
Marsha J. Dohrmann: 34, 36, 40, 46, 47, 53, 55, 56, 57, 66, 69L, 151. Walter Gasper: 164, 166T, 167R, 211L, 243. Craig Marshall: 11, 16L, 72, 78, 101, 110, 138, 155, 192, 206, 213. Stephanie McCann: 31, 33, 37, 39, 43, 45, 51. Tony Naganuma: 68, 98, 126, 177, and all Focus On, Health Career, Health Today, and Working Toward Wellness border graphics. Nelva B. Richardson: 87, 89, 90, 92, 95. Exercise Handbook: Sylvia Giblin: 249, 250, 251, 252, 253, 254, 255.

CONTENTS

9   Living in a Healthful Environment   218

TO THE STUDENT

You are learning to read because reading is an important skill. You are learning to do arithmetic problems because they are important skills, too. Learning about health can help you to be a healthy person. Having good health means that you can think, work, and play at your very best.

You should practice good health habits every day. They can help you to have the best possible health. The best possible health you can have is called *wellness.* Wellness is a goal that is reached by practicing good health habits every day.

HBJ Health offers you health information to help you make good decisions about your health. You can use this information to form good health habits. *HBJ Health* explains how different kinds of foods can help you grow to be a strong and healthy person. You will learn tips that you can use every day for playing safely. You will do certain activities to help you learn how rest, sleep, and exercise can help you reach wellness. You will learn ways that can help you enjoy your life without using harmful drugs.

HBJ Health encourages you to practice good health habits so you can enjoy your life to the fullest.

CHAPTER 1

Thinking About You

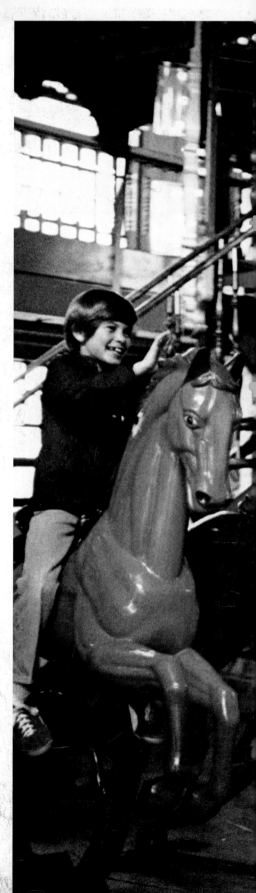

Have you ever wondered what makes you different from other people? Nobody else looks, thinks, feels, and acts exactly the way you do.

You are like other people in some ways, too. People all need the same basic things to stay alive and keep healthy. But the choices you make to meet your needs make you different from other people. For example, everyone needs food, yet you may not like the same foods as other people.

You share many other needs with other people. You may make different choices to meet your needs. The choices you make tell a lot about who you are.

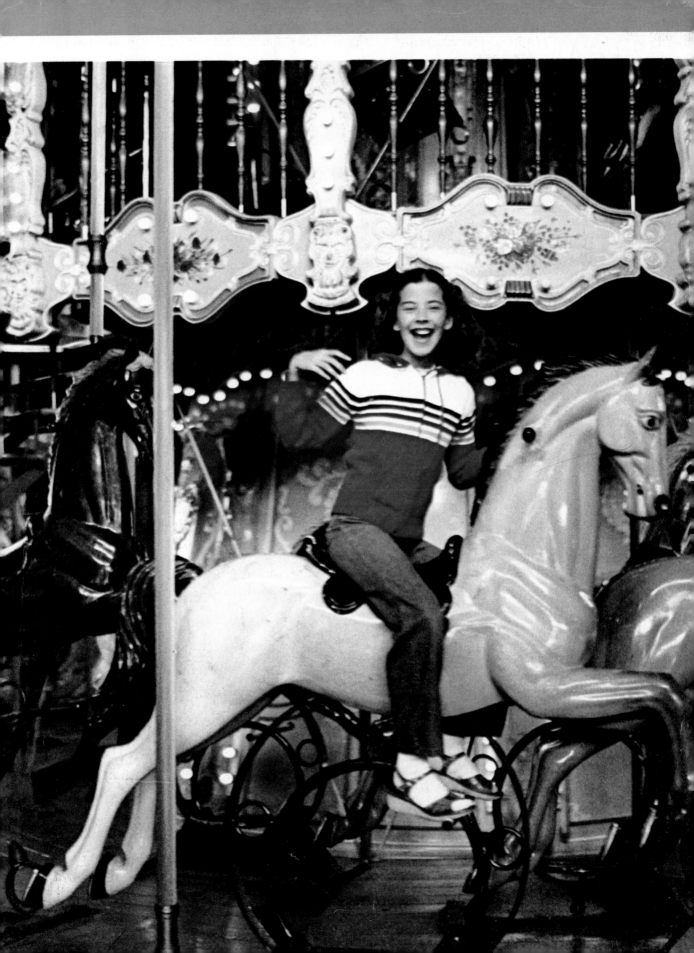

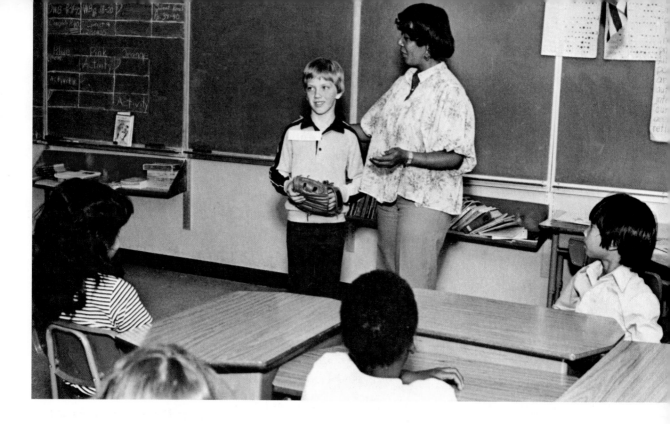

Victor is new in school. What might he be telling the class about himself?

WHAT MAKES YOU SPECIAL?

Today was Victor's first day at his new school. His teacher, Ms. Martinez, asked Victor to tell the class a little about himself.

"My name is Victor Gilman. I am nine years old. I have blond hair and blue eyes. My family just moved here from Fort Wayne, Indiana. I have an older brother and a younger sister. We have two dogs. I like playing baseball and reading books about baseball stars. I like roller-skating a lot, too. I'm teaching my sister how to skate."

Victor told many facts about himself that make him special. He told his name and age. He told what he looks like and what he likes to do. All these special features make him who he is. They make him different from anyone else. These features are some of Victor's **traits.** A trait is a feature that tells something about you.

Thinking About Your Traits

Think about some of your traits. Are you helpful, like Victor? Do you laugh a lot? Do you feel scared or sad sometimes?

You have your own special combination of traits. One of your traits is the way you look. Your size and shape are traits. Some other traits are the ways you feel and act. Your traits make you special.

Victor's class can see some of his traits. They can see that he is tall and thin. They can see his blond hair and blue eyes. But his class cannot see all of his traits. Victor has told the class some facts about these traits, too. He said that he is teaching his sister to skate. Being kind and helpful are two more of Victor's traits.

The ways you look, think, feel, and act are all traits. Taking good care of yourself can help keep these traits healthy. When your traits are at their best, you have **wellness**. Wellness is the highest level of health you can possibly reach.

Seeing Your Traits

Look into a mirror. What traits do you see? What color are your eyes? Your hair? Are you tall or short?

How is Victor being kind and helpful?

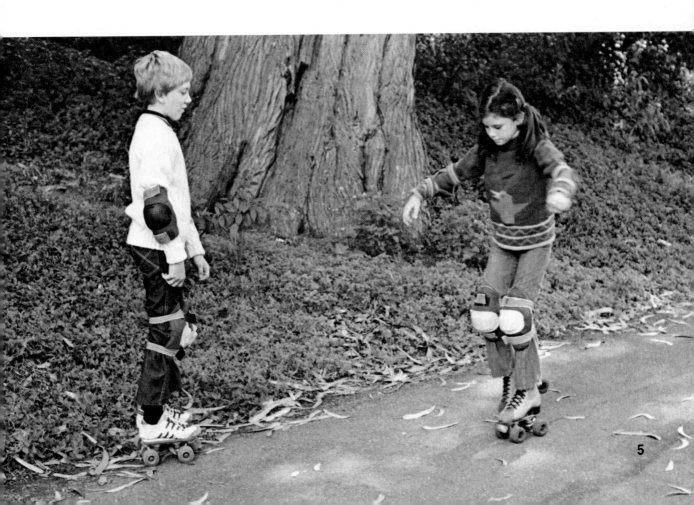

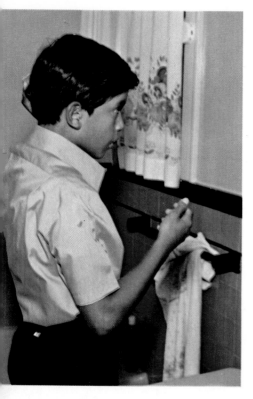

What kind of trait is Roberto's black hair?

The Way You Look

When Roberto looks into the mirror, he sees black hair and brown eyes. He sees someone who is short and thin. These are some of Roberto's **physical traits.** Physical traits are traits that tell about your body. Many of your physical traits can be seen in the way you look.

Roberto has other physical traits that he cannot see. The size of his lungs is a physical trait. The shape and size of his heart are physical traits, too. Even though Roberto cannot see these traits, they tell about his body.

Your physical traits tell about your body. You can see many of your physical traits when you look into the mirror. You can see the color of your eyes and hair. You can see how tall you are. You can see how you look.

The Way You Think About Yourself

The way you look does not tell only about your body. How you dress and whether you are neat are part of the way you look. Whether you smile or frown a lot is part of the way you look, too. These tell something about the way you think about yourself.

Some of your physical traits, like Roberto's, are hidden. The size of your heart is a physical trait. How well you see without glasses is a physical trait, too. Traits like these generally cannot be seen.

6

The Way You Think

Annette is very curious about plants and animals. She reads books about them and asks her science teacher many questions. Being curious is one of Annette's traits. It is part of the way she thinks.

Ron has a good imagination. He makes up stories about space travel and strange, new planets. Sometimes he likes to pretend that he is a character from a book. Ron's imagination is one of his traits.

The way you think is another of the traits that makes you special. Are you curious, like Annette, or imaginative, like Ron? Do you have a good memory? Can you learn things quickly?

What is one of Annette's traits? What is one of Ron's? How can you tell?

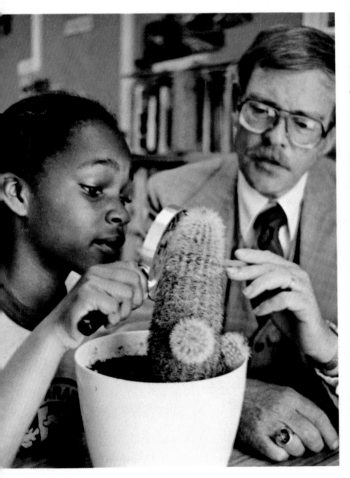

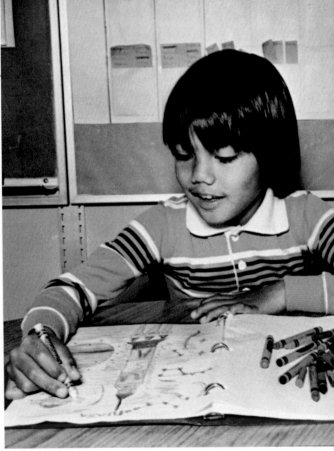

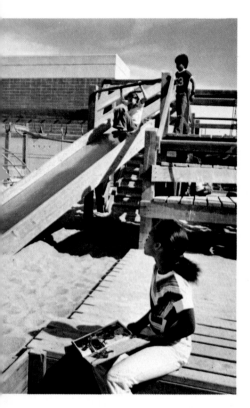

How might Annette be feeling? How can you tell?

The Way You Feel

Annette feels shy when she is around her classmates. She likes to sit alone and read most of the time. Ron is shy sometimes, too. He feels embarrassed about sharing his stories and games with other people.

Being shy is one way you can feel. It is a trait some people have. You can feel other ways, too. Some of the ways you can feel are happy, sad, excited, and proud.

The same situation can cause different people to feel different ways. That is because people have different traits.

Paula and Debbie were playing together at Debbie's house when a thunderstorm started. Paula felt afraid. One of her traits is fear of loud noises. But Debbie enjoyed watching the storm. Liking storms is one of Debbie's traits. The same storm made Paula feel frightened and made Debbie feel excited.

The Way You Act

Joe acts in different ways at different times. On the first day of school he was friendly to some new classmates. He wanted to make them feel welcome. He felt happy and excited. The next day he was not feeling well. Then he acted quietly and did not talk to people.

No one else acts exactly as you do. The way you act, like the way you feel, depends partly on your traits. It also depends partly on what is happening to you at the time. Joe is friendly most of the time. But he did not act friendly the day he did not feel well.

Thinking About How You Act

How do you usually act around other people? Are you often shy? Are you friendly to and interested in other people? Are you polite to others? Do you always act in the same way?

8

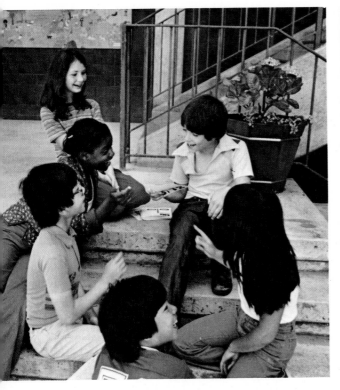
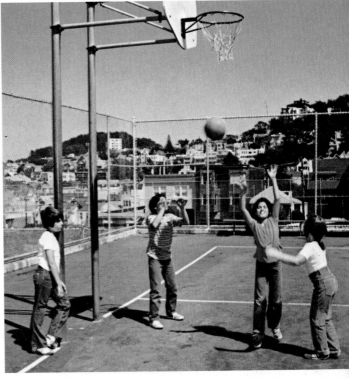

What are two different ways Joe is acting in these pictures?

Your Personality

The ways you look, think, feel, and act make up your **personality**. No one else has a personality that is just like yours. Your personality makes you the special person you are.

Your personality depends partly on traits you were born with. It also depends on things that have happened to you. And your personality depends on the choices you make to help yourself reach wellness.

REVIEW IT NOW

1. What is a trait?
2. What is wellness?
3. What are physical traits?
4. What is your personality?

School Counselor

Many schools have a *school counselor* to help students solve problems. Sometimes being in a new school is hard. Paying attention in class can be hard, too. And sometimes a student just needs to talk with someone. The school counselor is there to listen and to help. Often, a school counselor helps students make choices and decisions, too.

To be a school counselor, you need five years of college. You also may need a year of teaching. To learn more about being a school counselor, write to the American School Counselor Association, 5999 Stevenson Avenue, Alexandria, VA 22304.

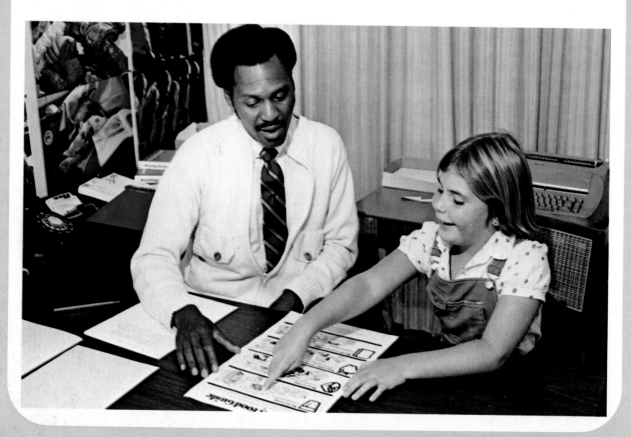

WHAT ARE PEOPLE'S NEEDS?

Your personality makes you different from everyone else. But in some important ways you are just like other people. One of these ways is your **needs.** A need is something that a person must meet or satisfy to be healthy. Everyone has the same basic needs.

Your Physical Needs

Sara and her classmates were discussing the things that everyone needs to stay healthy. Sara said that everyone needs food. Yim added that everyone needs water. Steve said that everyone needs to breathe air. Maria agreed with Steve. But she said that everyone needs to stay warm, too. So she added a place to live.

Food, water, air, and shelter are all things that your body needs to stay alive. They are **physical needs.** Everyone has the same physical needs.

Listing Ways to Find Shelter

Suppose a family lost their house in a fire or flood. How could they meet their physical need for shelter? List at least three things they might do.

What physical needs are shown here?

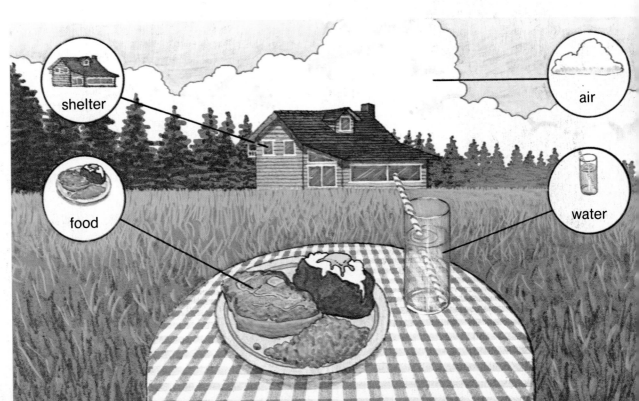

shelter

air

food

water

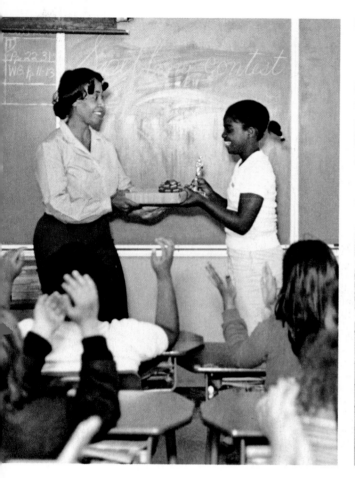

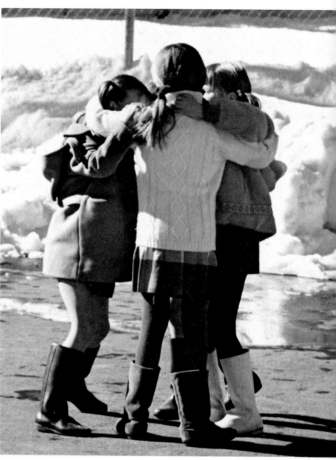

What emotional need has May satisfied? What emotional need have these children satisfied? How can you tell?

Thinking About Friendship

What traits might make someone a good friend? In what ways can a friend help you meet your emotional needs?

Your Emotional Needs

You have other needs, too. You need things that will make you feel good. You need to feel loved. You need to feel close to other people. You need to feel proud of yourself.

Needs that have to do with your feelings are **emotional needs.** Everyone has similar emotional needs.

May has won first prize in the school spelling contest. Her prize makes her feel proud of herself. That is one of her emotional needs.

The children who are playing together feel close to each other. Feeling close is an emotional need.

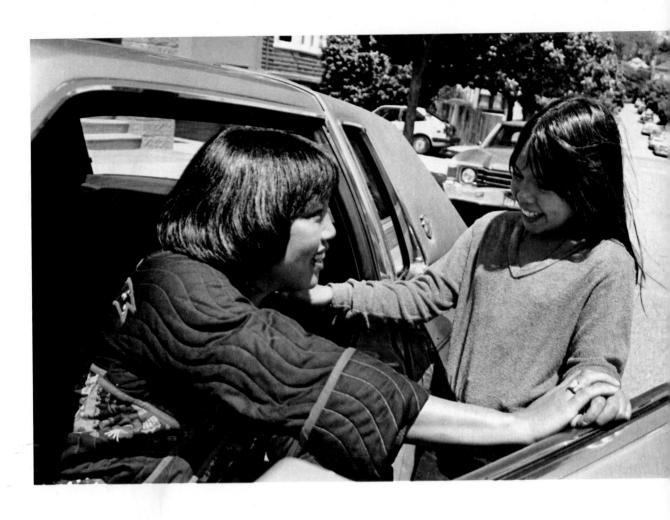

Linda likes to be with her Aunt Deborah. They talk about many things and go places together. Aunt Deborah makes Linda feel loved. Feeling loved is another emotional need.

How might Linda be feeling? How can you tell?

You can stay alive without meeting your emotional needs. But you probably will not be happy. When you are not happy, your body may not be as healthy as it should be.

REVIEW IT NOW

1. What are physical needs?
2. What are emotional needs?

Taking Charge Over Anger

Health Today

What do you do when you are angry? Showing anger can cause problems when you say or do something you do not really mean. But "hiding" anger will not work either. Just like joy and sadness, anger is a feeling. Everyone feels angry at some time. If you hold anger in, it can grow stronger.

The next time you begin to feel angry, take charge over it. Sometimes it helps to talk. Sometimes it helps to take a deep breath and count to 20 before acting. It may help to bounce a ball or take a walk, too. Taking charge over your anger can help you stay happy—and healthy.

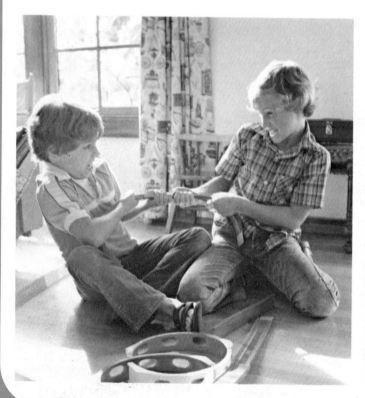
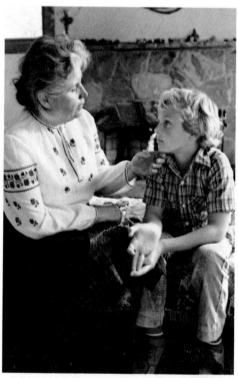

HOW CAN YOU MEET YOUR NEEDS?

What can you do if your needs are not being met? Sometimes you can change the way you look, think, or feel. Sometimes you can meet your needs by changing your actions. You can do something that makes you feel good about yourself. Then you can meet the need to be proud of yourself. You can be more friendly. That can bring you closer to others and satisfy another need.

Thinking About Yourself

Amy liked to watch television. But that kept her from doing her homework. Sometimes her work was messy or late. Then she could not feel proud of herself. She felt angry with herself all the time.

What might Amy do to feel better about herself and her homework?

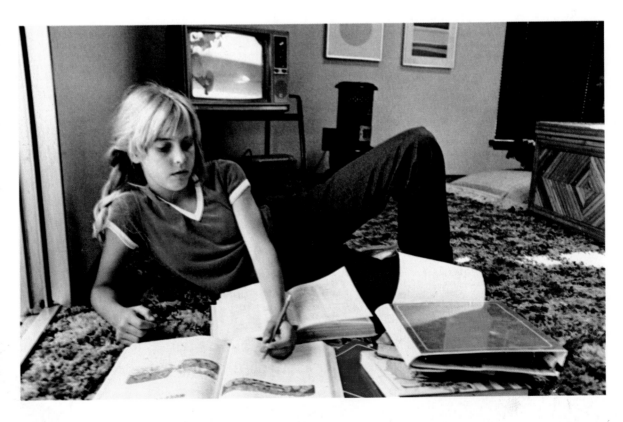

WHAT I LIKE ABOUT MYSELF

1. I keep my room neat.
2. I try to be fair in games
3. I do not give up easily.

WHAT I WOULD LIKE TO CHANGE

1. Get homework done earlier.
2. Practice the piano.
3. Make more friends.
4. Take better care of my garden.

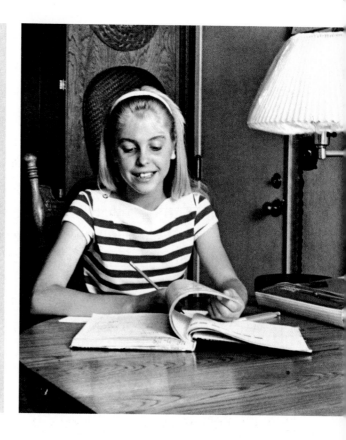

Look at Amy's list. What change might she have made to feel better about herself and her homework?

Amy decided to do something to change the way she felt. She thought about herself for a while. Then she made two lists. One list showed things about herself that she liked and did not want to change. The other list showed things about herself that she wanted to change.

Amy started watching less television. That gave her more time for homework, so her work was always neat and on time. She also had more time to practice the piano. She spent more time in her garden. And she made some new friends.

Amy has changed her way of acting. Her new actions have changed her way of feeling. Now she is not angry with herself all the time. By changing some of her actions, Amy helped satisfy her need to feel proud of herself.

Knowing Your Strengths and Weaknesses

Sometimes you have to find out what you do well and what you do not do so well in order to meet your needs. You have to know your own strengths and weaknesses.

Merrie is honest with herself about ballet. She knows she will never be a great dancer. But she practices every day because she enjoys dancing. She knows it makes her look and feel good. Practicing every day makes Merrie feel good about herself.

Both Amy and Merrie were honest with themselves. That means they knew their strengths and their weaknesses. Both girls worked to change themselves. They satisfied their need to feel proud of themselves.

Talking About Strengths

With a friend or a classmate, list some strengths people might have. Talk about how each could make a person feel.

How might practicing ballet every day help Merrie feel good about herself?

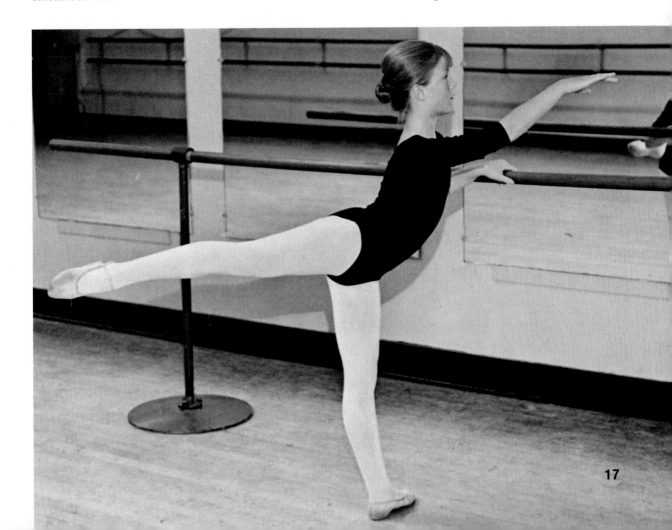

Arlene Blum

Arlene Blum is a famous mountain climber. In 1978, she led a team of women to the top of a mountain called Annapurna. They were the first Americans to reach the top of Annapurna. In 1980, Arlene led eight women up another mountain called Bhrigupanth. No one had ever climbed Bhrigupanth before Arlene and her team.

Arlene had to know her strengths and weaknesses in order to climb both mountains. She had to trust that her strengths would help her succeed. Arlene did succeed. And she was proud of herself and her team.

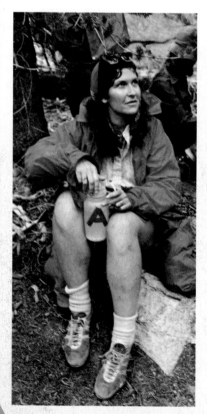
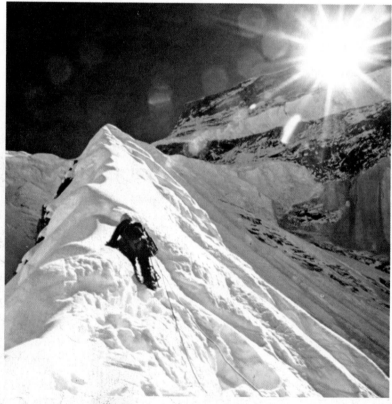

Making Choices

You can change the way you act in some ways. Sometimes you can change the way you look, feel, or think. But you have some traits that cannot change. You cannot always make the changes you want to. You may have to make choices to satisfy your needs in other ways.

Martin is doing some things he enjoys. Martin would like to do other things, too. He would like to ride a bicycle and ice-skate. But Martin cannot do these things. That is because he was born with a heart that does not work as it should.

Martin cannot change this physical trait. He cannot do everything he would like to do. But he has learned to do some things well. He spends time doing what he enjoys. He enjoys building models and teaching his friends how to build them.

Martin has chosen ways to act that make him feel good about himself and bring him close to other people. Martin's choices help him meet his needs.

Thinking About Making Choices

Think about a time when you had to make a choice to satisfy a need. What was the choice you made? When did you make the choice? What need did you satisfy?

How might Martin be meeting his emotional need to feel close to others?

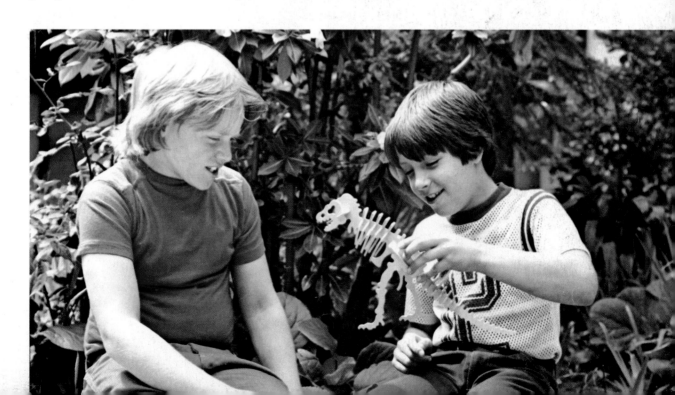

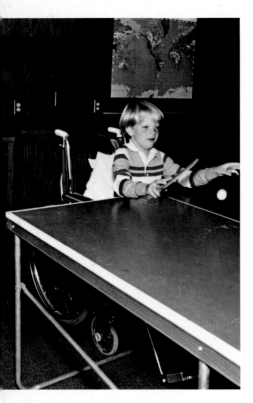

How can choosing to be cheerful help Max feel good about himself?

Making Healthful Choices

Some traits can make it hard for you to do everything you want to do. But you can do some of the things you want. And you can satisfy your needs for love and closeness. You can make choices that help keep you healthy.

Max cannot walk by himself. But there are many things he can do. He can swim and play Ping-Pong. He can do magic tricks. He can tell jokes. Max has chosen to be cheerful about what he can do. He has chosen to do these things well. His choices make him feel good about himself. They make other people feel good about him, too. He has many friends. Max has chosen ways to take care of his needs. He realizes that these choices will help him reach wellness.

Everyone has some traits that cannot be changed. Probably you will never be able to do all of the things you want to do. But you can do some things to satisfy your needs. In many ways, you can decide how to look, think, feel, and act. These choices will help you be the healthiest person you can be.

REVIEW IT NOW

---

1. What is one example of something you can do if your needs are not being met?
2. What need can making changes help you meet?
3. What is an example of a trait that cannot be changed?

Recognizing Personality Traits

Here is a personality activity you can do with your friends or family.

Give a piece of paper and pencil to each player. Have the players write three personality traits about themselves. These traits should be ones that another person cannot "see." For example, "like sports," "love dogs," and "interested in music" are personality traits.

Put the pieces of paper into a bowl. Have one player at a time choose a paper and read the three traits aloud. The other players guess whose personality the paper describes.

How well do others know you?

Working Toward Wellness

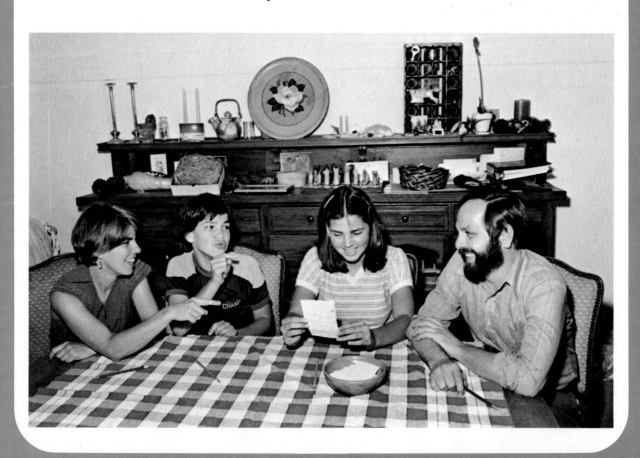

To Help You Review

Checking Your Understanding

Write the numbers from 1 to 11 on your paper. After each number, write the answer to the question or questions. Page numbers in ( ) tell you where to look in the chapter if you need help.

1. What are four kinds of traits that make a person different from anyone else? (**5**)
2. What kind of physical trait is the size of a person's lungs? (**6**)
3. What are four different ways of feeling? (**8**)
4. Why do people sometimes feel different ways in the same situation? (**8**)
5. What are three things a person's personality depends on? (**9**)
6. Which kind of needs must people meet to stay alive? (**11**)
7. What are four different physical needs that everyone has? (**11**)
8. What are three different emotional needs that everyone has? (**12–13**)
9. What can a person do if his or her needs are not being met? (**15**)
10. What are strengths? What are weaknesses? (**17**)
11. What might a person have to do if he or she has a trait that cannot change? (**19**)

Checking Your Health Vocabulary

Write the numbers from 1 to 7 on your paper. After each number, write the letter of the meaning for the word or words. Page numbers in ( ) tell you where to look in the chapter if you need help.

1. trait (4)
2. wellness (5)
3. physical traits (6)
4. personality (9)
5. needs (11)
6. physical needs (11)
7. emotional needs (12)

a. things a person must meet or satisfy to be healthy
b. the ways you look, think, feel, and act
c. needs that have to do with your feelings
d. a feature that tells something about you
e. things your body needs to stay alive
f. the highest level of health you can possibly reach
g. traits that tell about your body

Each of the words below describes a feeling. Write the numbers from 8 to 13 on your paper. After each number, write a sentence using each word.

8. shy
9. happy
10. sad
11. excited
12. proud
13. afraid

Practice Test

True or False?

Write the numbers from 1 to 15 on your paper. After each number write *T* if the sentence is *true*. Write *F* if it is *false*. Rewrite each false sentence to make it true.

1. All of your traits can be seen by other people.
2. No one else has a combination of traits exactly like yours.
3. Your physical traits tell about the way you act.
4. Being curious is a trait that is part of the way a person thinks.
5. The same situation can cause different people to feel different ways.
6. The way you act depends only on the traits you were born with.
7. Some of your friends can have personalities just like yours.
8. Your personality depends partly on things that have happened to you.
9. Needs your body must meet to stay alive are emotional needs.
10. Not everyone has the same basic physical needs.
11. Everyone has different emotional needs.
12. When you are not happy, your body may not be as healthy as it should be.
13. Sometimes you can meet your needs by changing your actions.
14. You never can change the way you look, feel, or think.
15. Sometimes people must make choices to satisfy their needs in healthful ways.

Complete the Sentence

Write the numbers from 16 to 20 on your paper. After each number, copy the sentence and fill in the missing word.

16. Your hair color and eye color are examples of _____ traits.
17. Your personality is the way you look, think, feel, and _____.
18. _____, water, air, and shelter are things your body needs to stay alive.
19. The need to feel loved is an _____ need.
20. Part of being honest with yourself is knowing your strengths and _____.

24

Learning More

For You to Do

1. Draw a picture of yourself. Show at least four of your physical traits. Show some of your personality traits, too. For example, if you like animals, you might draw yourself holding a cat or dog.

2. Choose one of the people described below. Write down what the person's two most important physical needs and two most important emotional needs might be.
   - an astronaut going to the moon alone
   - a child lost on a mountain in a storm
   - a boy or girl going to a new school
   - a boy or girl who is having trouble with schoolwork

For You to Find Out

1. Why do children often have the same physical traits as their parents? How is the information that is turned into physical traits passed on to the children? To find out, look for library books about *heredity*.

2. What are twins? How are *identical* twins different from *fraternal* twins? Which kind of twin is more likely to have physical traits that are the same? Do twins have similar personality traits, too? Use an encyclopedia to find out about twins.

3. Many people have had to live with different kinds of physical traits that keep them from doing certain things. One person is Roy Campanella, who was once a famous baseball player. Find out about Roy Campanella. How did he learn to live with his physical trait? What choices did he have to make in order to start a new career?

For You to Read

Here are some books you can look for in your school or public library to find out more about your personality and your needs.

Booher, Dianna D. *Making Friends With Yourself & Other Strangers*. Messner, 1982.

Swenson, Judy H. *No One Like Me*. Dillon Press, 1985.

CHAPTER 2

What Is Your Body Like?

There is more to you than meets the eye. Under your skin is a world you never get to see. It is a world of muscles, bones, blood, pumps, tubes, and many other kinds of parts. All these parts are controlled by your brain.

The world outside your body is full of things to see, hear, touch, smell, and taste. The world within your body helps you know the world outside. Your brain and all the other parts of your body work together to help you live. Keeping these body parts healthy requires special effort. Your job is to practice good health habits to help yourself reach wellness.

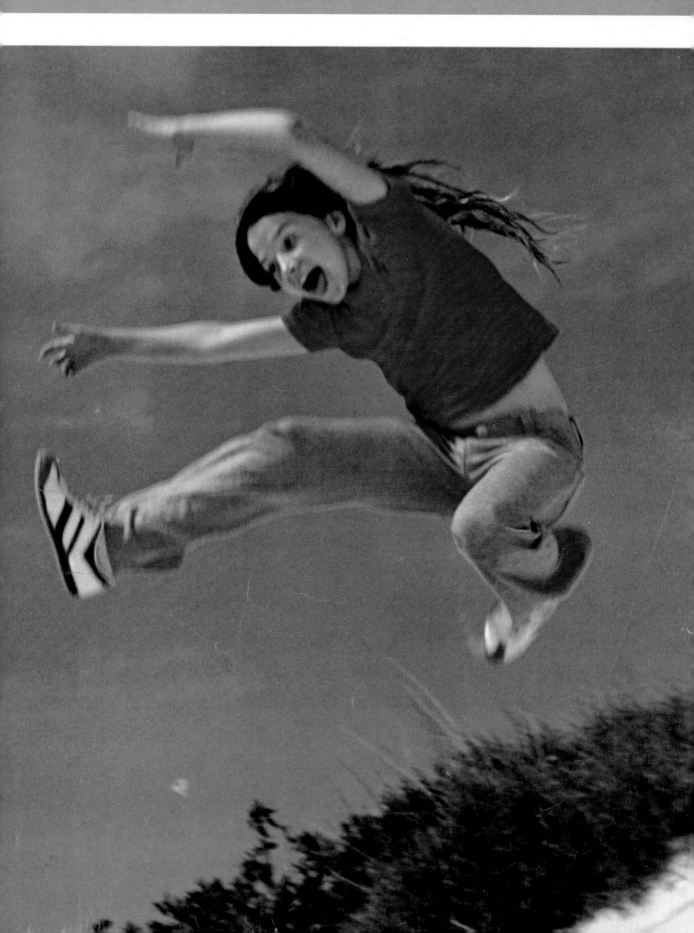

ABOUT YOUR BODY

Your body is made up of many different parts. Each part of your body does a certain job. Some parts work by themselves. Other parts work together. But each part of your body, no matter how small, has a job to do. When all the parts of your body work as they should, you are healthy.

Your Cells

Your skin, bones, muscles, and blood are all parts of your body. But each is made of smaller parts. The smallest living parts of your body are called **cells.**

Cells are the building blocks of your body. Every part of your body is made of cells. Your bones are made of bone cells. Your skin is made of skin cells. Your whole body is made up of many kinds of tiny, living cells.

One cell is too small to see with only your eyes. Hundreds of cells would fit on the head of a pin. You can see a cell if you look at it through a **microscope.** A microscope makes small things look bigger.

Finding Out About Cells

About how many cells are in the human body? You might look in an encyclopedia to find the answer.

Look at the pictures of bone cells, nerve cells, and muscle cells. In what ways are these cells different?

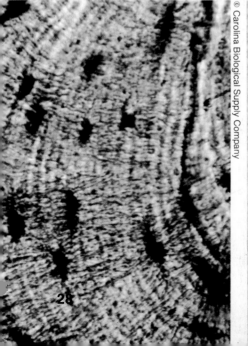
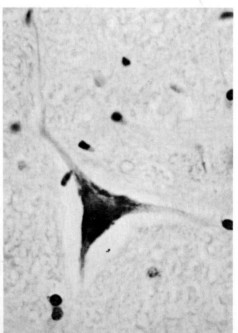
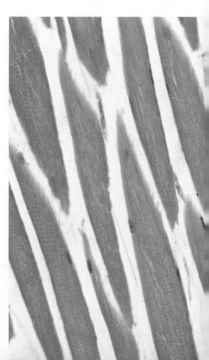

© Carolina Biological Supply Company

28

Rodney is looking through a microscope to see some cells. The cells are from the inside of his cheek. The round picture shows what Rodney sees. He would see something different if he looked at bone cells. Skin cells, bone cells, and other kinds of cells look different from one another. They do different jobs, too.

Your Tissues

Cells that look alike work together to do the same job. Skin cells, for example, are round and flat. They fit together tightly. The cells work together to cover and protect your body. Your skin is made of many skin cells working together.

Groups of the same kinds of cells working together are **tissues.** Skin is one kind of tissue in your body. Bones and muscles are two other kinds of tissues. Your body is made up of many kinds of tissue.

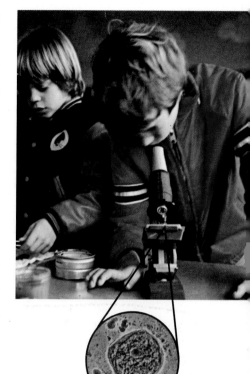

How does the microscope help Rodney see the cells?

What is the muscle tissue made of? the nerve tissue? the skin tissue?

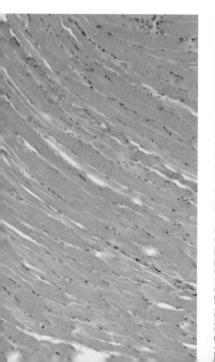
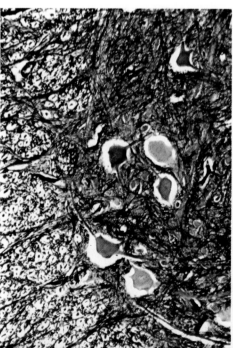
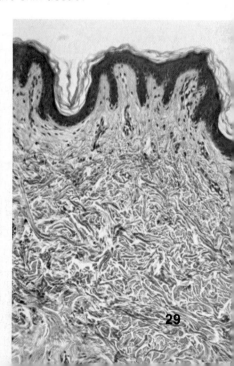

29

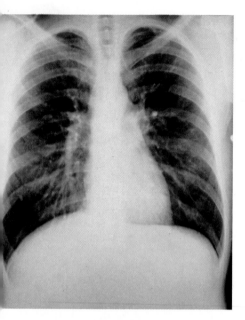

An X-ray shows organs and other parts inside the body.

Your Organs

Tissues in your body also work together in groups. Groups of tissues that work together are **organs.** Each organ does a certain job. Your heart is an organ. It has the job of pumping your blood. Like all organs, it is made up of several kinds of tissue. Your stomach, your brain, and your eyes are some of your other organs.

Your Body Systems

Your organs help you do the things you need to do to stay alive and healthy. You need to eat and breathe. You need to move and think. You need to understand the world around you. Each of your organs helps with one of these jobs. But no organ does the whole job by itself. Several organs work together to meet each of your body's needs.

Organs working together make up a **body system.** Different body systems take care of different needs. For example, one body system helps you breathe. Another body system helps you move around.

Every body system has several organs. For example, your nose is an organ of the system that helps you breathe. Your lungs are other organs of the same system. The organs do different jobs to help the whole system work.

The chart shows the body systems you will read about in this chapter. It also shows the jobs these systems do. Your body systems work together to keep you healthy.

About Your Body

The **appendix** is an organ in your body that does not have any job. But the appendix can become infected. When it is infected, it can burst open. Poisons can enter the body and make a person very ill.

BODY SYSTEMS

Skeletal System

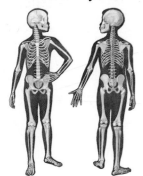

Gives your body shape

Muscular System

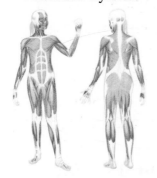

Helps your body move

Digestive System

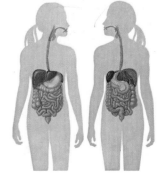

Breaks up food for your cells to use

Respiratory System

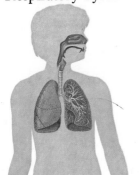

Helps your body breathe

Circulatory System

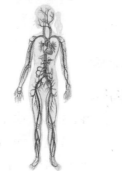

Carries food and other things to your cells

Nervous System

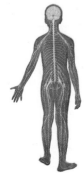

Controls all the other systems in your body

What is the job of each body system shown here?

REVIEW IT NOW

1. What are the smallest living parts of your body?
2. What are tissues?
3. What is a group of tissues working together called?
4. What is a body system?

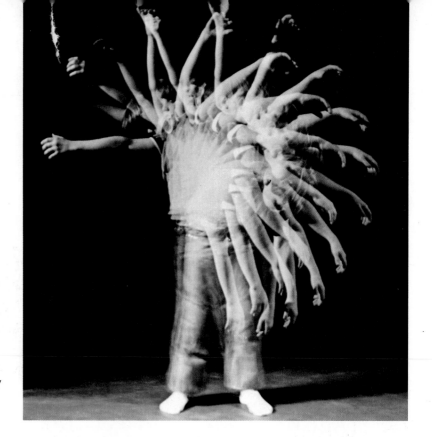

Try moving your arms as many ways as you can. What kinds of movements can you make?

HOW DOES YOUR BODY MOVE?

Look at your hand. You can move your hand in many ways. You can swing your thumb all around and curl all your fingers. Many other parts of your body can bend, twist, and move, too.

Two body systems help you move the way you do. One is your **skeletal system.** It gives your body its basic shape. The other system is your **muscular system.** It helps your body move.

Your Skeletal System

All of the bones in your body make up your skeletal system, or **skeleton.** Your skeleton makes your body firm and gives it shape. Without your skeleton, your body would be soft, like a caterpillar. Because you have a skeleton, you can stand up. You can sit, walk, or run without losing your shape.

Finding Out About Bones

How many bones do you have in your body? You might use an encyclopedia to help you find out.

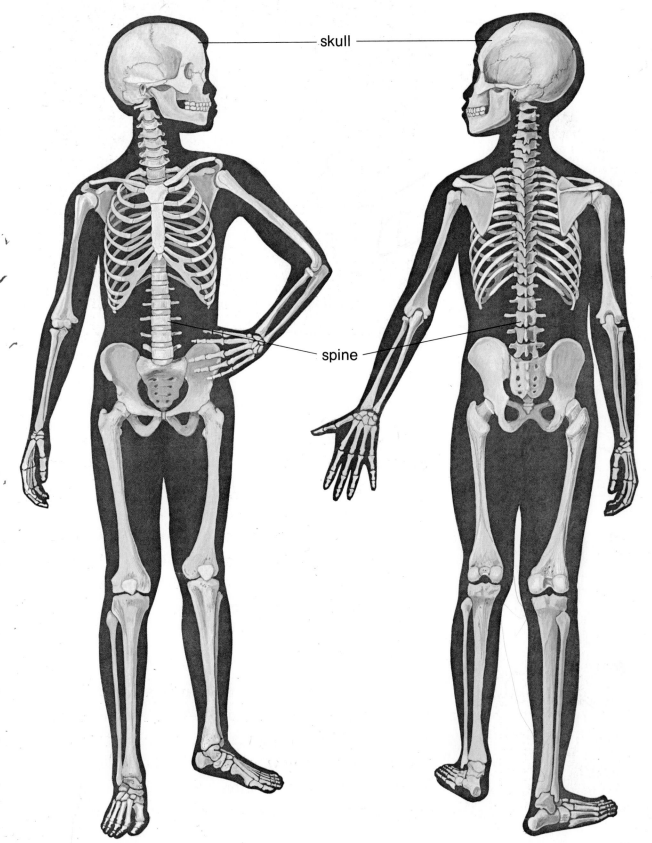

skull

spine

Where in your body do you have a hinge joint? a ball-and-socket joint? immovable joints?

Bones are stiff, like pencils. They cannot bend. But your body can bend in many places because your skeleton is made of many bones. Your body can bend in places where bones connect. These places are called **joints.** Your skeleton has many joints.

One kind of joint swings open and shut like a door on a hinge. This kind is a **hinge joint.** Your elbow is a hinge joint.

Another kind of joint lets one bone move in a circle. This is a **ball-and-socket joint.** The end of one bone is round. It fits into a cup-shaped place on another bone. Your hip is a ball-and-socket joint. It lets your leg swing all around.

Some joints do not let your bones move. These are **immovable joints.** A rounded set of bones called your **skull** covers your brain. These bones do not move. Their job is to protect your brain from being hurt. If these bones moved, they could not do their job.

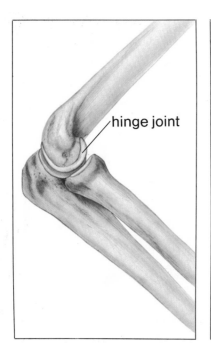

hinge joint

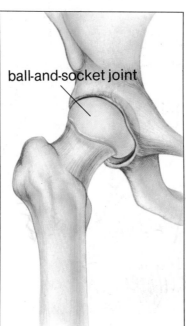

ball-and-socket joint

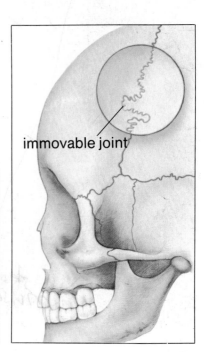

immovable joint

X-ray Technician

If you have ever had an X-ray, it probably was taken by an *X-ray technician.* The technician operates the X-ray machine.

X-ray photographs show doctors the heart, bones, lungs, and blood. These photographs often help doctors find out what might be wrong with a person. Doctors then can decide on the treatment a person might need.

X-ray technicians take special training programs after high school. These programs usually last from two to four years. To learn more about being an X-ray technician, write to the American Society of Radiologic Technologists, 15000 Central Avenue SE, Albuquerque, NM 87123.

Health Career

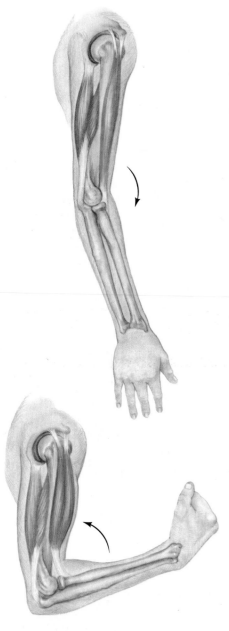

Your Muscular System

Your bones can move only with the help of your muscular system. **Muscles** are the organs of your muscular system. They attach to bones and other parts of your body to help them move. For example, some muscles move your eyes as you read. Other muscles make up some of the organs of your body systems. Your stomach, for example, is made of muscle.

Muscles move some parts of your body by pulling on your bones. They move your legs by pulling your leg bones. They move your fingers by pulling your finger bones.

Muscles cannot push. They can only pull. But muscles work in pairs to move your bones and other parts of your body. For example, two different muscles move your elbow. One muscle pulls the bones of your lower arm up to make your elbow bend. Another muscle pulls the same bones down to make your elbow straighten.

Your bones and muscles help you run, walk, and play. They help you every time you move any part of your body.

What did the arm muscles do to cause the arm to bend?

REVIEW IT NOW

1. What two body systems help you move?
2. What does your skeleton do?
3. What are three kinds of joints in your skeleton?
4. How do muscles move parts of your body?

36

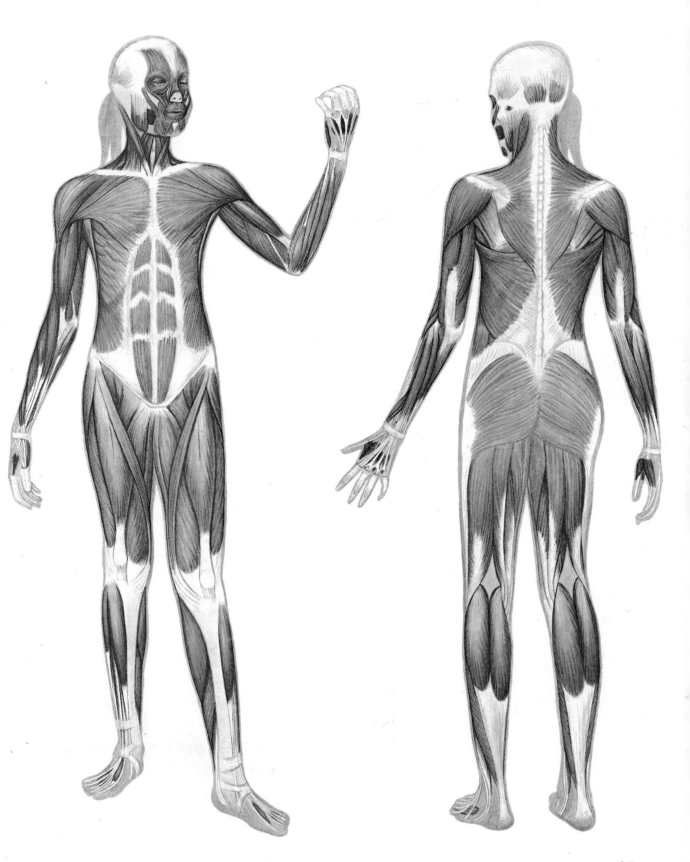

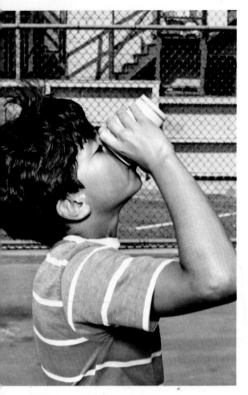

Which body system will change the juice into materials this boy's cells can use?

WHAT HAPPENS TO THE FOOD YOU EAT?

Every day you probably drink milk, water, or fruit juice. You probably eat meat, bread, and many other foods. Your cells need materials in food in order to do their work. Without them, your cells die.

The materials in the food you eat go to all your cells. But first the food must be broken into tiny pieces. Then it can be changed into materials that your cells need to stay alive. The breaking up and changing of your food is called **digestion.** The body system that breaks up and changes your food is your **digestive system.**

Your Digestive System

Several organs make up your digestive system. A few of them are solid. But most of these organs are hollow tubes. The tubes are connected end to end. Food moves from one tube to the next. Each organ pushes the food to make it move. Some of the organs of the digestive system make special liquids called **digestive juices** that help digest food.

When you eat, you put food into your mouth. Your teeth begin breaking your food into smaller pieces as you chew. Then you swallow. Your food passes into your **esophagus.** The esophagus is a tube made of muscle. It squeezes food down into your body, the way you might squeeze toothpaste out of a tube.

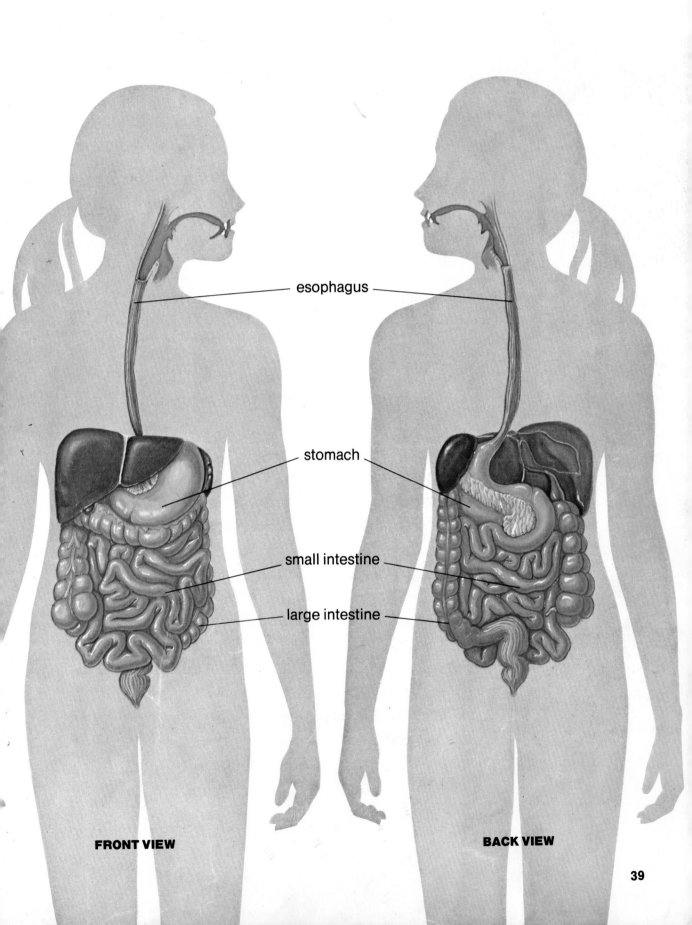

esophagus

stomach

small intestine

large intestine

FRONT VIEW

BACK VIEW

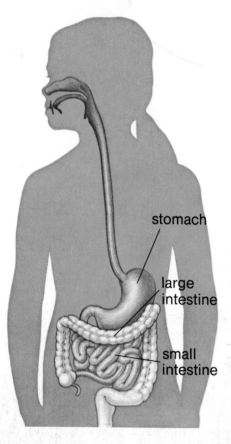

stomach

large intestine

small intestine

What organs of the digestive system are shown here?

Your esophagus pushes the food down into your **stomach.** Your stomach is like a sack with openings at both ends. Its walls are made of muscles. These muscles squeeze and mash up your food. Digestive juices help break up your food, too. Most food stays in your stomach for a few hours.

When food leaves your stomach, it passes into your **small intestine.** Your small intestine is filled with digestive juices. Most digestion takes place in the small intestine.

Your small intestine is only as wide as a finger. But it is about 13 feet (4 m) long in someone your age. That is more than twice as tall as you are! It is all curled up inside your body. From your small intestine, the materials in the digested food go to your cells.

The food you eat has many parts that your body cannot digest or use. Materials that your body cannot use are called **wastes.** These wastes move into your **large intestine.** Your large intestine is wider and shorter than the small intestine. It is nearly 4 feet (1.2 m) long. Wastes are stored in the large intestine until they leave your body.

REVIEW IT NOW

1. What is digestion?
2. Where does digestion begin?
3. What does your esophagus do?
4. Where does most digestion take place?
5. What organ stores wastes until they leave your body?

WHAT HAPPENS TO THE AIR YOU BREATHE?

Suppose you are playing outdoors. You run fast. You bend and twist your body. Soon you are breathing hard. When you stop playing and rest, your breathing slows down. But it never stops. You have to keep breathing all the time to stay alive.

You must breathe because your cells need a gas called **oxygen.** They need oxygen in order to use food materials. You get oxygen from the air you breathe. Your **respiratory system** controls your breathing. It helps you get the oxygen you need. It also gets rid of a gas called **carbon dioxide.** Carbon dioxide is a gas your cells make but cannot use.

As these girls run fast, do they breathe in more or less oxygen than when they rest?

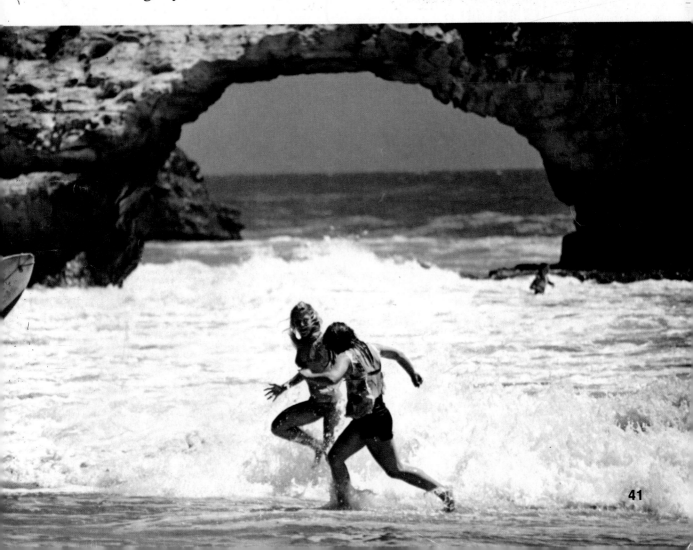

41

Your Respiratory System

The air you breathe enters your body through your nose. Some air may also enter through your mouth. Your nose warms up the air that enters it. Tiny hairs inside your nose remove some of the dust and dirt from the air.

The air then moves into a tube called the **windpipe.** This tube goes from your nose and mouth down into your chest. There your windpipe branches into two parts. One branch goes into each of your two **lungs.** Your lungs are large organs inside your chest.

Your lungs contain thousands of tiny **air sacs** that are like small balloons. They fill with air when you breathe in. They take the oxygen out of the air and send it to all your cells. At the same time, carbon dioxide moves into the air sacs. Your cells make carbon dioxide. The carbon dioxide leaves your body when you breathe out.

Finding Out About Iron Lungs

What is an iron lung? In what way does it help a person breathe? For what illness were iron lungs mainly used? You might use library books or an encyclopedia to help you find out.

REVIEW IT NOW

1. What do your cells need in order to use food materials?
2. What does your respiratory system do?
3. How does air get from your nose to your lungs?
4. What moves into the air sacs when oxygen leaves them?

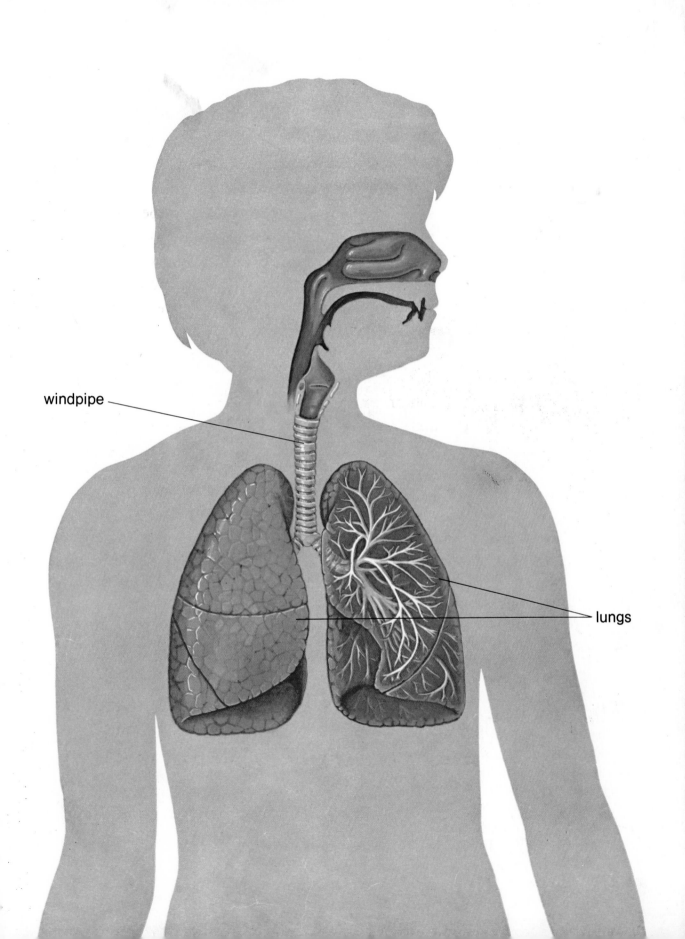

windpipe

lungs

HOW DO FOOD AND OXYGEN GET TO YOUR CELLS?

Look at your feet. They are far away from your small intestine and from your lungs. But the cells in your feet need materials in food and oxygen to stay alive. Food materials and oxygen must be carried to all your cells. Your **circulatory system** does this important job. The same system carries wastes away from each cell. Wastes are things the cells make and cannot use. All cells have to get rid of their wastes.

What are the three types of blood cells your blood contains?

Your Circulatory System

Your circulatory system is made up of three main parts. Your **blood** carries food and oxygen to your cells. It also carries away their wastes. Your **heart** pumps your blood and keeps it moving all the time. Your **blood vessels** are small tubes that carry the blood to and from all parts of your body.

Your blood moves through your body without stopping. Most of your blood is a clear liquid. In fact, most of your blood is water. Your blood also has cells floating in it.

You have three types of blood cells. **Red blood cells** are tiny, round cells. Their job is to carry oxygen to all your cells. **Platelets** are another type of blood cell. They help form a scab when you cut yourself. **White blood cells** help your body fight certain kinds of illness by attacking **microbes.** Microbes are tiny living creatures that can make you ill if enough of them get inside your body.

blood vessels

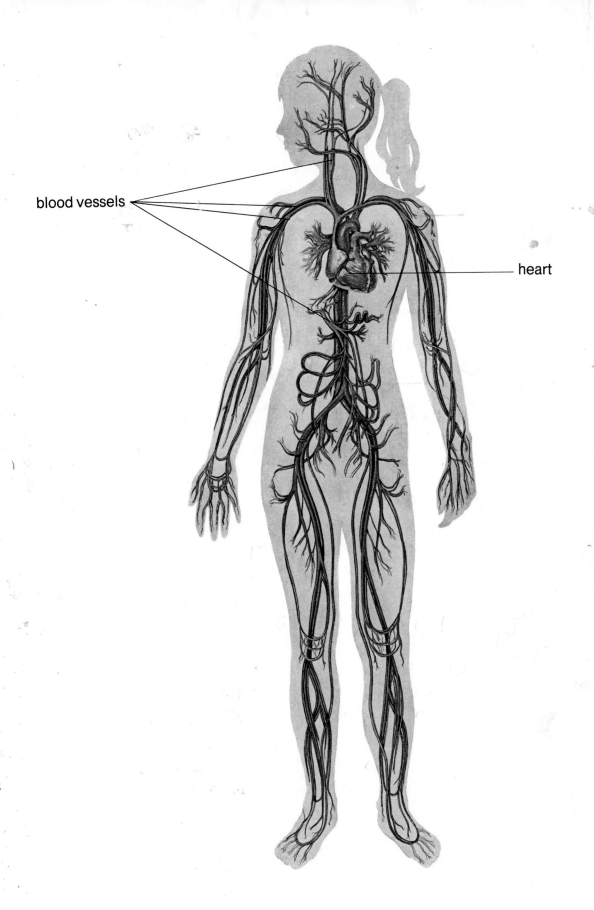

heart

Which blood vessels carry blood away from the heart? Which carry blood back to the heart?

Your heart is a hollow organ made of muscle. It is about the size of your fist. Your heart works by filling up with blood. Then it squeezes the blood into your blood vessels. The squeezing is called your **heartbeat.** Your heart beats about once a second when you are resting. It beats faster when you move and work hard.

You have three kinds of blood vessels. **Arteries** carry blood away from your heart. **Veins** carry blood back to your heart. You also have millions of very tiny blood vessels called **capillaries.** Capillaries connect arteries to veins.

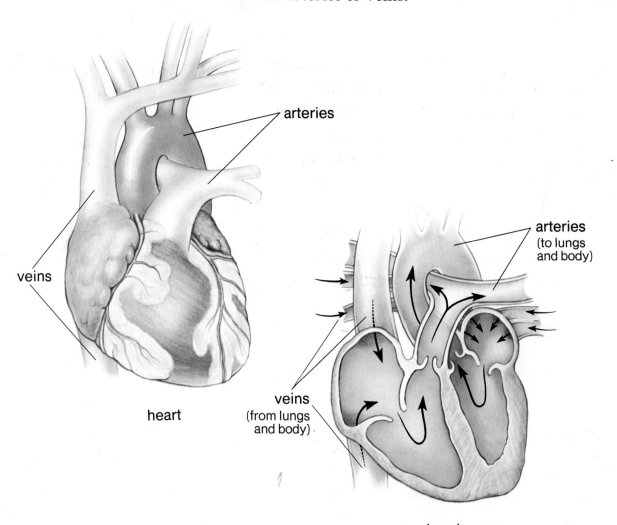

arteries

veins

heart

arteries
(to lungs and body)

veins
(from lungs and body)

heart

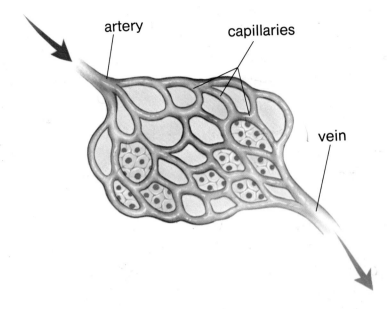

artery

capillaries

vein

What moves into the cells through the capillary walls? What moves out of the cells through the capillary walls to be carried away?

Capillaries have thin walls. Food materials and oxygen can move right through the walls. Capillaries in your small intestine let food materials into your blood. Capillaries in your lungs let oxygen into your blood. Capillaries near your cells let the food materials and oxygen out of your blood and into your cells. Capillaries also carry away wastes from your cells. Every cell in your body has a capillary near it.

Your circulatory system helps keep your cells alive. It brings your cells everything they need and takes away wastes that your cells cannot use.

Blood Vessels in Your Body

You have about 62,000 miles (100,000 km) of blood vessels in your body.

REVIEW IT NOW

1. What does your circulatory system do?
2. What are the three main parts of the circulatory system?
3. What are the three types of blood cells?
4. What are the three kinds of blood vessels?

Arthur Ashe

Focus On

Arthur Ashe's name is known to most people who enjoy tennis. Twice he was a championship winner. But late in 1979, his career, and his life, almost came to an end. He had a heart attack.

Arthur Ashe always worked very hard to be a winner. He was fit and strong. It came as a surprise to him that he could have heart trouble. But his health and strength probably helped save his life.

Since his heart attack, Arthur Ashe has changed his life-style. He has worked slowly and carefully to gain back his health and strength. He knows staying healthy and strong is important all of a person's life.

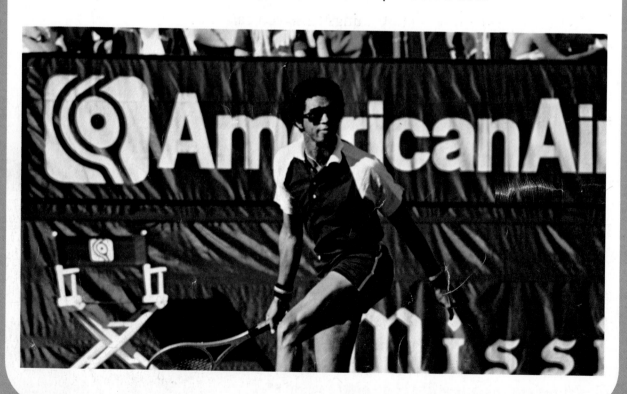

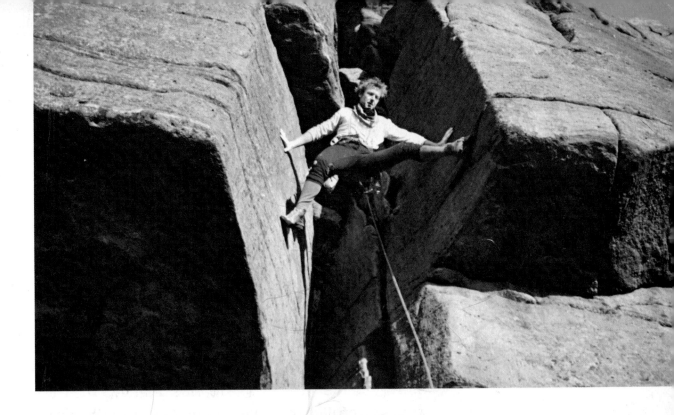

WHAT MAKES THE PARTS OF YOUR BODY WORK TOGETHER?

Your body does many more things than you can count. It does more than the biggest and best machine in the world. One system in your body controls the many things that you do. It is your **nervous system.**

Your Nervous System

Your nervous system is made up of three main parts. All of the parts of your nervous system are made of special cells called **nerve cells.**

Your **brain** tells every other part of your body what to do. It is the organ that you use to think.

The brain is like several computers all working at once. It is a busy message center. It receives messages from all over your body. It sends messages to all parts of your body, too.

Which organ of the nervous system tells the mountain climber's body what to do?

Finding Out About Your Brain

Find out the names of at least three parts of your brain. What is the main job of each? You might use library books to help you find out.

49

**Thinking About the
Spinal Cord**

Suppose a person's
spinal cord is damaged.
What might happen?

Messages travel to and from your brain through **nerves.** Nerves are bundles of long nerve cells. They connect all parts of your body with your brain. Some nerves, such as those in parts of your face, connect directly to your brain. Other nerves connect to your brain through a large bundle of nerves called the **spinal cord.**

Your spinal cord goes down the center of your back. The top of your spinal cord is connected to your brain. Your spinal cord is soft. It is protected by a stack of bones called your **spine.** Some people call it the "backbone."

Nerves branch out from your spinal cord and go to many parts of your body. They go to your arms, chest, legs, and feet. These nerves carry messages from the brain through the spinal cord. The messages tell these parts how to work. Nerves also carry messages back to the brain through the spinal cord, telling the brain what each part is doing.

Your brain, spinal cord, and nerves work together. They make you able to do all the things that you do. They help you move. They help you see, hear, smell, and taste. They help you learn and think. They make every part of your body work the way it should.

REVIEW IT NOW

1. What body system controls everything you do?
2. What are the main parts of your nervous system?
3. How do messages travel to and from your brain?
4. What is your spinal cord?

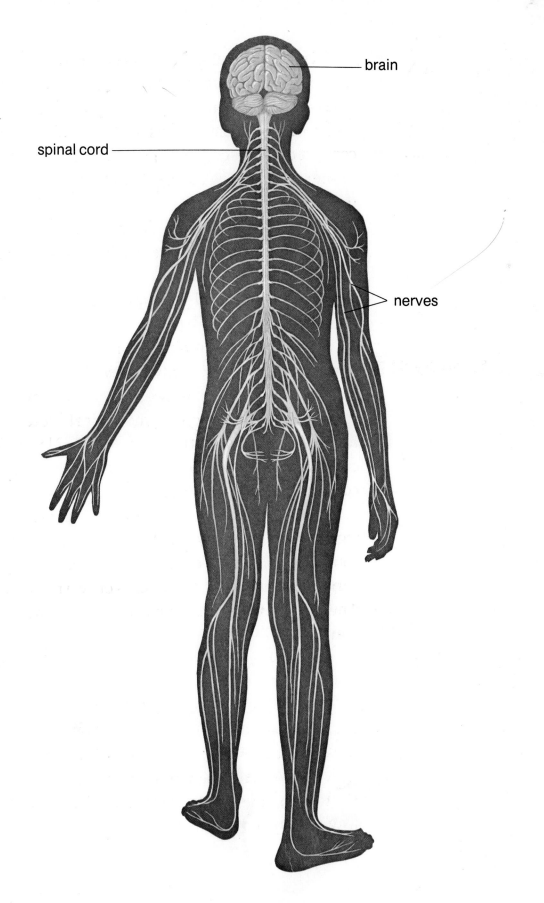

brain

spinal cord

nerves

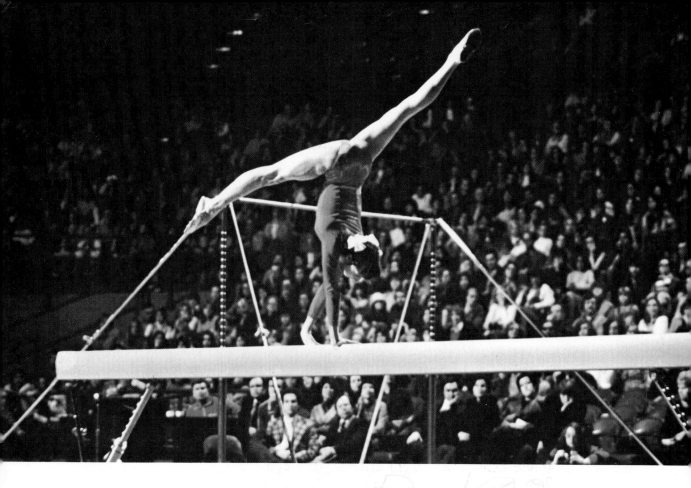

Your senses help you keep your balance.

ABOUT YOUR SENSES

What can you tell about the world around you at this moment? You can see the other children in your class. You can hear the sounds around you. You can read what is written on this page. You know if your classroom is too hot or too cold.

You find out about the world around you through your **senses.** Your five major senses are seeing, hearing, smelling, tasting, and touching. Each of your senses picks up messages from outside and inside your body. Each can **sense,** or become aware of, certain information about the world. For example, your ears can sense sounds. They work with your nervous system to help you hear. None of your senses can work without your nervous system.

Your Other Senses

You also have some other senses that tell about your body. One of these is your sense of balance. It helps you keep from falling over. Another is your sense of hunger. It tells your body when you need food to eat.

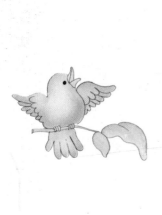

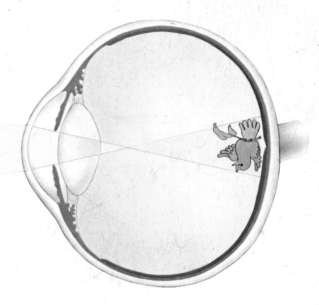

Your Eyes and Your Sense of Seeing

Your eye works much like a camera. It makes an upside-down picture of what you see.

Your eyes work with your nervous system to help you see. You see only when light enters your eyes. The light makes a little picture inside your eyes. It makes a picture of whatever you are looking at.

Look at the drawing of the eye. You can see that it has many different parts. Light passes through all the parts of your eye. When light reaches the nerves at the back of your eye, it makes a little picture. Your nerves take messages about the picture to your brain. Your brain figures out what the messages mean.

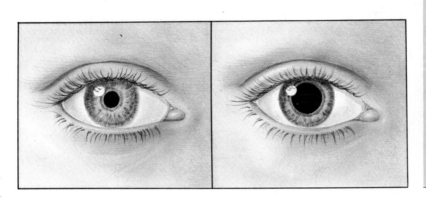

Your Pupils

Your pupils control how much light enters your eyes. Your pupils are large in dim light. The large size lets as much light as possible into your eyes. In very bright light, your pupils are very small. Very little light enters your eyes.

The Sonic Guide

Health Today

Many blind people use special aids to help them walk. Now there is a new aid called the *Sonic Guide.*

The Sonic Guide is attached to a pair of eyeglasses. It is wired to send beeps into the blind person's ears. The beeps let the person know that there is an object nearby. They also signal whether the object is near or far, or whether it is on the right or left of the person. The Sonic Guide even signals whether the object is rough or smooth.

People who are blind and also cannot hear can use the Sonic Guide, too. These people cannot "hear" the beep, but can "feel" it instead.

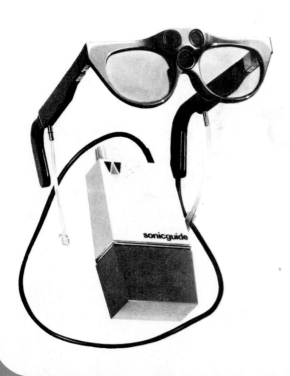

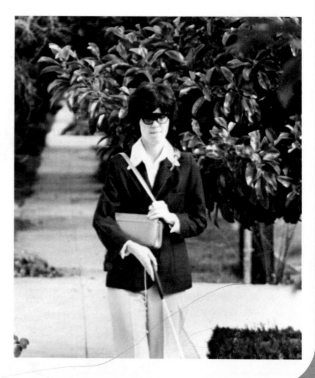

Your Ears and Your Sense of Hearing

Your ears work with your nervous system to help you hear. Nerves in your ears pick up messages about sounds. Sounds are caused by air moving in a certain way. Anything that makes a sound makes air move in this way.

The moving air enters your **outer ear.** This is the part of your ear that people can see. You hear with your **inner ear.** Your inner ear is inside your head.

The drawing shows the three main parts of your ear. When the moving air enters your ear, it makes some parts move. Nerves in your inner ear take messages about the movement to your brain. Your brain figures out what the messages mean.

Talking Without Sound

Say something to a friend or classmate without making any sound. Just move your lips. Can your friend tell what you said?

You hear with which part of your ear?

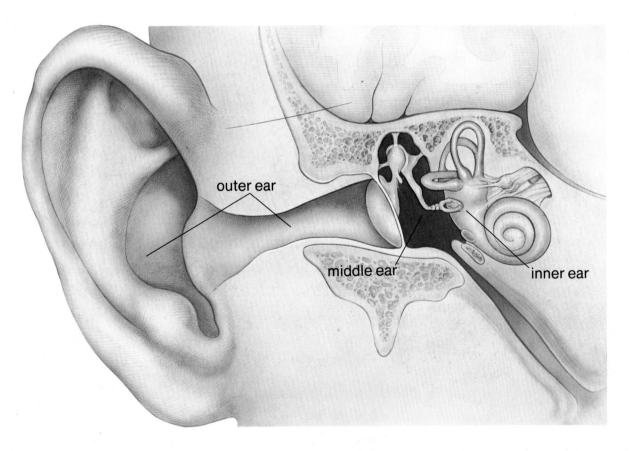

outer ear

middle ear

inner ear

Your Nose and Your Sense of Smell

When you breathe, your nose takes in air. Often, smells, or **odors,** enter your nose, too. Special nerve cells in your nose pick up these odors. They take messages about the odors to your brain. Then you know what you are smelling.

Your nose has another job, too. It works with your tongue to help you taste food.

Your Tongue and Your Sense of Taste

Your tongue is covered with hundreds of little bumps. These bumps contain your **taste buds.** Each taste bud has a nerve cell in it. The nerve cells can identify the tastes of food. They send messages about the tastes to your brain.

Most foods also have odors. When you chew, nerve cells in the back of your nose pick up the food odors. These cells send messages to your brain, too. But what you taste is really a mixture of taste and smell.

Your Skin and Your Sense of Touch

Your skin gives you your sense of touch. It contains millions of special nerve cells. These cells let you know certain things about objects that you touch. Some nerve cells can tell if an object is cold. Other nerve cells can identify heat. Some cells identify pain. Your skin can tell if something is rough or smooth, hard or soft.

Your senses help keep you alive. They help you enjoy life, too.

odors

Bumps on the tongue contain your taste buds.
Which senses work together to help you taste food?

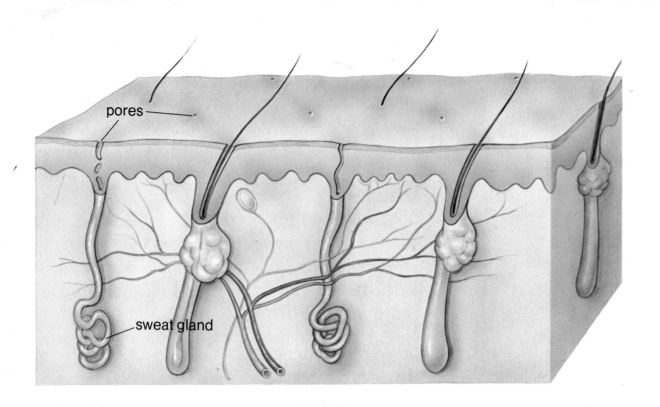

pores

sweat gland

Another Job of Your Skin

Your skin has many different jobs. One important job is to help control your body temperature. **Sweat glands** in your skin produce a liquid waste called **sweat.** Sweat leaves your skin through small openings called **pores.** When the sweat dries, it cools your skin. It lowers your body temperature.

How might your skin also protect you from harmful microbes?

REVIEW IT NOW

1. What are your five major senses?
2. What do your eyes need in order to see?
3. What part of your ear do you hear with?
4. What two senses work together when you taste food?
5. What sense does your skin give you?

Working Toward Wellness

Testing Your Sense of Touch

Try this activity with your family or friends and test your sense of touch.

Find a box with a top. Cut a hole that is large enough for a hand to reach into the box. Fill the box with several objects from inside and outside your home. The objects might include an apple, a comb, a bar of soap, a rock, or a shell. Be careful to use objects that are not sharp and that will not harm the skin.

Have your family or friends each take a turn. With eyes closed, reach into the box and pick up one object. Describe the object by how it feels. Write down the words the person uses to describe it. Who can guess what the object is?

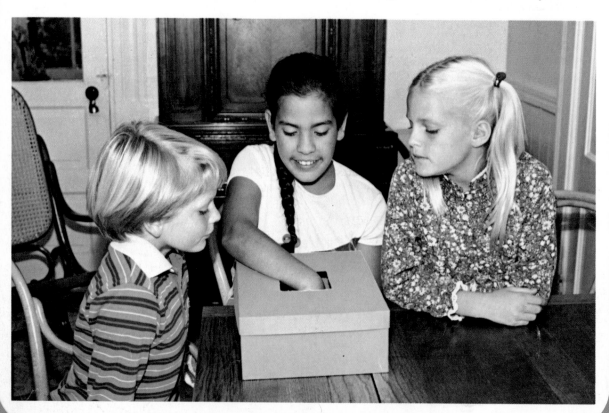

To Help You Review

Checking Your Understanding

Write the numbers from 1 to 14 on your paper. After each number, write the answer to the question or questions. Page numbers in ( ) tell you where to look in the chapter if you need help.

1. Where in your body do you have a hinge joint? Where do you have a ball-and-socket joint? (**34**)
2. What set of bones in your body contains immovable joints? (**34**)
3. What must happen to the food you eat before it can go to your cells? (**38**)
4. What gas do you breathe in? What gas do you breath out? (**41**)
5. What do red blood cells do? What do white blood cells do? What do platelets do? (**44**)
6. What is the squeezing of your heart called? (**46**)
7. What organ might you call the "message center" of your body? (**49**)
8. What protects your spinal cord? (**50**)
9. What is the job of the nerves that branch out from your spinal cord? (**50**)
10. What are your five major senses? (**52**)
11. Why is it impossible to see something in a room that is totally dark? (**53**)
12. What causes the sounds you hear? (**55**)
13. With what part of your ear do you hear? (**55**)
14. What does your skin contain that gives you your sense of touch? (**56**)

Checking Your Health Vocabulary

Write the numbers from 1 to 10 on your paper. After each number, write the letter of the meaning for the word or words. Page numbers in ( ) tell you where to look in the chapter if you need help.

1. cells (28)
2. tissues (29)
3. organs (30)
4. body system (30)
5. skeletal system (32)
6. muscular system (32)
7. digestive system (38)
8. respiratory system (41)
9. circulatory system (44)
10. nervous system (49)

a. organs working together on the same job
b. body system that carries food and oxygen to all your cells and takes away wastes
c. groups of alike cells working together
d. body system that gives you your basic shape
e. groups of tissues working together
f. body system that controls the many things you do
g. smallest living parts of your body
h. body system that breaks up your food
i. body system that helps you breathe
j. body system that helps you move

Write the numbers from 11 to 16 on your paper. Then write a sentence that explains the meaning of each word or words. Page numbers in ( ) tell you where to look in the chapter if you need help.

11. skeleton (32)
12. muscles (36)
13. digestion (38)
14. wastes (40)
15. microbes (44)
16. outer ear (55)

Write the numbers from 17 to 26 on your paper. After each number, write the letter of the meaning for the word or words. Page numbers in ( ) tell you where to look in the chapter if you need help.

17. joints (**34**)
18. esophagus (**38**)
19. stomach (**40**)
20. small intestine (**40**)
21. large intestine (**40**)

22. windpipe (**42**)
23. lungs (**42**)
24. air sacs (**42**)
25. nerve cells (**49**)
26. nerves (**50**)

k. the organ that squeezes and mashes up food
l. large organs inside your chest
m. places in your body where bones connect
n. special cells that make up your nervous system
o. the tube that squeezes food down into your stomach
p. the organ where most digestion takes place
q. tiny balloonlike sacs in your lungs
r. bundles of long nerve cells
s. the organ that stores wastes from food
t. the tube from your nose and mouth down into your chest

Write the numbers from 27 to 32 on your paper. Then write a sentence that explains the meaning of each word or words. Page numbers in ( ) tell you where to look in the chapter if you need help.

27. blood (**44**)
28. heart (**44**)
29. blood vessels (**44**)

30. arteries (**46**)
31. veins (**46**)
32. capillaries (**46**)

Practice Test

True or False?

Write the numbers from 1 to 15 on your paper. After each number, write *T* if the sentence is *true*. Write *F* if it is *false*. Rewrite each false sentence to make it true.

1. All organs are made up of only one kind of tissue.
2. Your bones can bend.
3. Muscles can pull and push your bones.
4. Most of the organs in your digestive system are hollow tubes.
5. Digestive juices help digest food.
6. Most digestion takes place in your stomach.
7. Your breathing and heartbeat slow down when you rest.
8. Most of your blood is a clear liquid.
9. Your nerves carry messages between your brain and all the parts of your body.
10. Your spinal cord is a stack of bones.
11. All of your senses work without your nervous system.
12. You can see only when light enters your eyes.
13. You hear with your outer ear.
14. Your taste buds can identify odors.
15. Nerve cells in your skin can identify pain.

Complete the Sentence

Write the numbers from 16 to 20 on your paper. After each number, copy the sentence and fill in the missing word.

16. _____ are the building blocks of your body.
17. Your _____ makes your body firm and gives it shape.
18. Your stomach walls and esophagus are made of _____.
19. Your cells need food materials and _____ to stay alive.
20. Your five major senses are seeing, hearing, _____, tasting, and touching.

Learning More

For You to Do

1. Digestive juices contain *acids* that help you digest food. Vinegar is an acid, too. Soak several kinds of food in vinegar for a day. Use a piece of meat, bread, and a green vegetable. How does each kind of food change? Which kind of food might someone digest most easily?

2. Blindfold a friend. Ask your friend to hold his or her nose. Feed your friend a slice of an apple and a slice of an onion. Can your friend tell which is which? Now have your friend blindfold you. Try the test yourself. Which senses do you need in order to taste food?

For You to Find Out

1. Find out the names of at least five organs in your body. To which body system does each organ belong? Library books about body systems might be a source of this information.

2. What does a fish heart look like? What does a snake heart look like? A lion's heart? Use library books or an encyclopedia to find out what each looks like.

3. What does a nerve cell look like? In what way does its shape help it carry messages? Look in an encyclopedia to find out more about nerve cells.

4. How sharp is a dog's sense of smell? How do dogs use their sense of smell? What animals besides dogs have a sharp sense of smell? An animal doctor might be able to answer your questions.

5. Why is the eardrum a delicate part of the ear? How deep is it inside the ear? How can it be protected from injury? Library books about the human body may help you answer these questions.

For You to Read

Here are some books you can look for in your school or public library to find out more about your body.

Bruun, Ruth, and Bruun, Bertel. *The Human Body*. Random House, 1982.

Sharp, Pat. *Brain Power: Secrets of a Winning Team*. Lothrop, Lee & Shepard Books, 1984.

Silverstein, Alvin, and Silverstein, Virginia. *The Story of Your Mouth*. Coward-McCann, 1984.

CHAPTER 3

Food for Growth

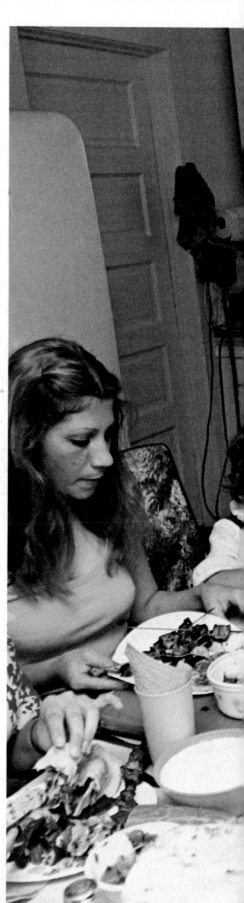

You may not have noticed, but you are probably taller now than you were last year. There are also many other ways you are growing. But you usually do not notice your own growth happening.

Your body needs different kinds of food to help it grow. You may have heard someone say, "Eat all you want." But the foods that you want may not always be the foods that you need. Eating the right foods will help you grow properly. The best food choices for you are the ones that will help you reach wellness.

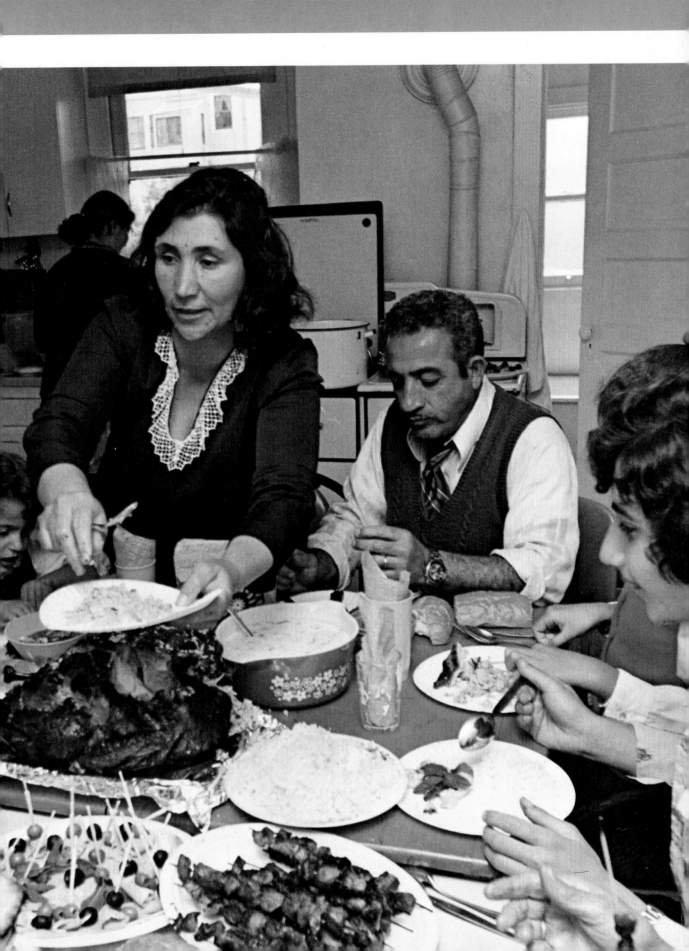

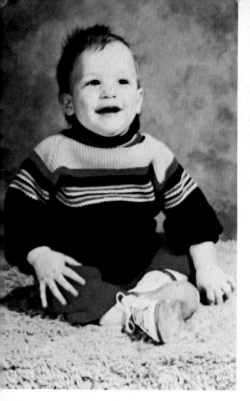

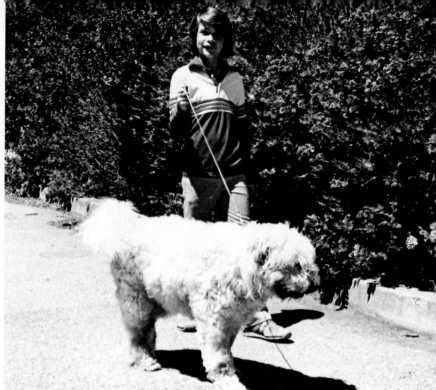

HOW YOUR BODY GROWS

Look at these pictures of Clifford. The one on the left was taken nine years ago. Clifford was tiny then. He was much smaller than the family dog. The picture on the right shows what Clifford looks like now. He has grown so much that now he can walk the dog.

You may not notice yourself growing from day to day. But you have grown a lot since birth—and you are still growing.

Your body gains size by making more and more cells. Your body grew from one small cell. It was smaller than a grain of salt. Then your one cell turned into two cells. Your two cells became four cells. The four became eight. The eight became sixteen. None of your cells grew any bigger than that first cell. But your cells kept increasing in number.

How does one cell become two? two become four? four become eight?

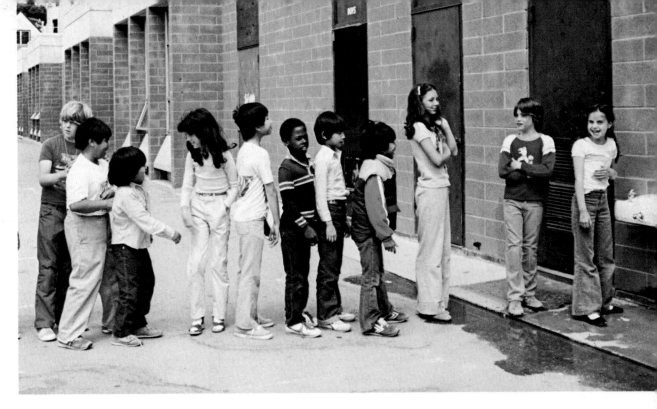

Now you have more cells than you can count. And your body is making new cells all the time. Parts of your body, such as your hair and nails, make new cells all your life.

What differences do you see in the heights of Clifford and his classmates?

How Fast You and Others Grow

Look at the picture of Clifford and some of his classmates. All the students are about the same age. Yet they are not all the same size. Some are taller and some are shorter. The shapes of their bodies are different, too.

Differences like these are normal at any age. People grow in different ways. Faye grew faster than Phyllis last year. But Phyllis may catch up with Faye this year. No one grows at the same speed all the time.

Growth follows a pattern, however. People grow quickly at certain times. At other times they grow more slowly.

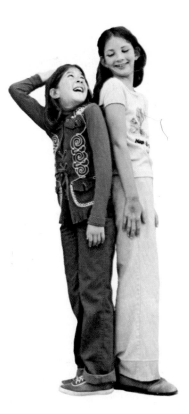

HEIGHT AND AGE

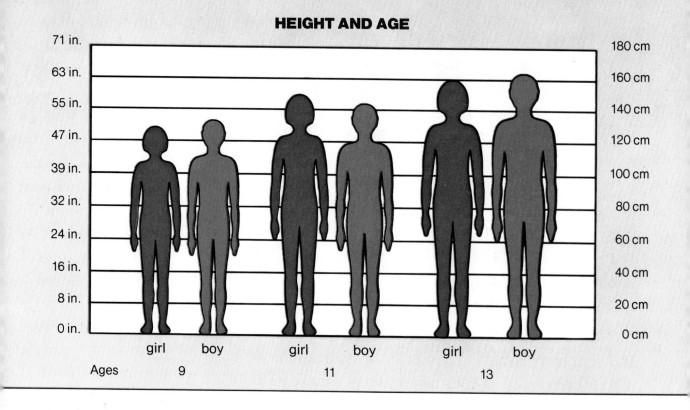

girl	boy	girl	boy	girl	boy

Ages 9 11 13

Some girls and boys may be taller or shorter than the figures in the chart. Why is this so?

Look at the chart. It shows the pattern of growth for girls and boys. The growth pattern is a little different for girls than for boys. At your age, for example, girls often begin growing faster than boys. Girls usually are taller than boys around the age of 11 or 12. Then growth begins to slow down in most girls. It speeds up in many boys. Within a few years, most boys are taller than most girls.

REVIEW IT NOW

1. How does your body grow in size?
2. Until what age are most girls taller than most boys?

Looking at Growth in Bones

By looking at X-ray pictures of hand and wrist bones, doctors can tell how quickly or slowly a young person's bones are developing.

When babies are born, their wrist bones are not very hard. They cannot be seen on X-rays. But as babies grow older, their bones grow bigger, harder, and closer together. They can be seen on X-rays. If X-rays show that the wrist bones are growing the way they should, the same probably is true of other bones in the young person's body.

Doctors also can look at X-ray photographs of the knee and the teeth to tell how a young person's bones are developing.

Health Today

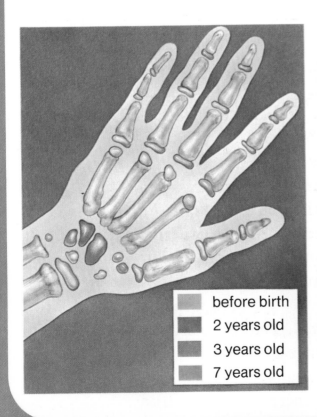

before birth
2 years old
3 years old
7 years old

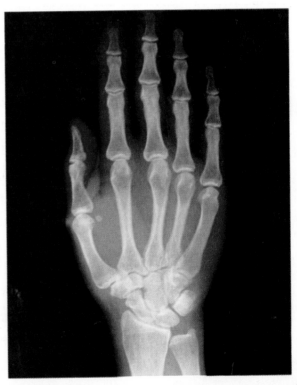

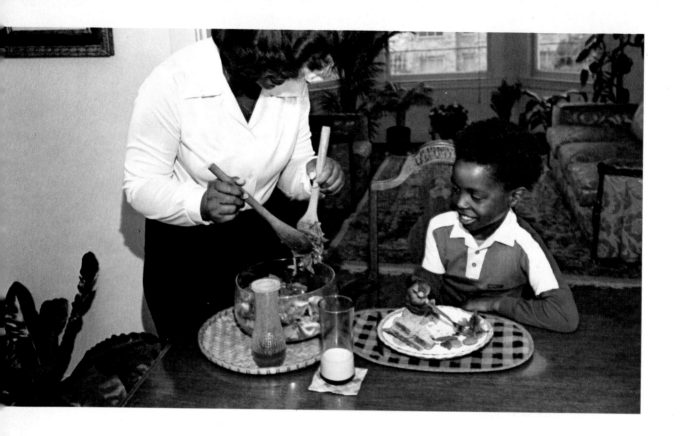

Why might Daniel need to eat a lot of food lately?

FOOD TO HELP YOU GROW

Daniel Walker has been eating a lot of food lately. Mrs. Walker knows that Daniel is growing, so she makes sure that he gets all the food he needs.

What Do You Need for Growth?

Like Daniel, you are growing. You need food for growth. Your body grows by making new cells. It has to have materials from which to make the new cells. These materials come from food.

You also need food to get energy. Any work you do takes energy. You use energy to play, to study, and even to sleep. You need energy to make new cells, too. The parts of food that help your body grow and give you energy are **nutrients.**

70

Velda de la Garza

Velda de la Garza knows about nutrition and health. She is a clinical dietitian in a hospital in Houston, Texas.

Often, very sick people lose their appetites and stop eating. Their bodies become weak and they lose too much weight. Velda helps decide the best way to feed a person and provide the nutritional needs that can strengthen the body.

Velda knows the importance of nutrition for a strong body. She says that nutrition is something that can be controlled. With her help, a person sometimes can regain strength in two or three days.

Focus On

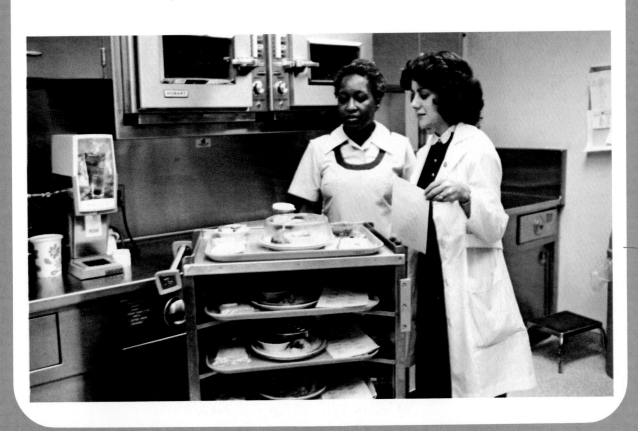

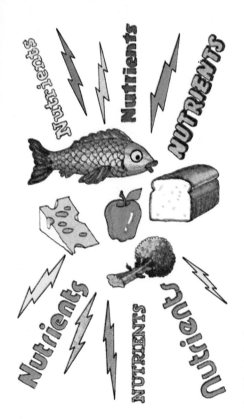

Why do you need to eat many different kinds of food?

Thinking About Your Favorite Food

What is your favorite food? What kind of nutrients does it have? What might happen if you ate only that food?

Nutrients You Need

Your body needs many kinds of nutrients. No one food has them all. To stay healthy, you must eat many different kinds of food.

Some foods give you nutrients for growth. They help build your muscles. Fish, beans, eggs, milk, cheese, and lean meat have plenty of these nutrients.

Some foods give you nutrients to use for energy. Sweet foods, bread, rice, noodles, fruit, and potatoes give you energy that you can use right away.

Another nutrient gives you energy that you can store. Most meats have some of this nutrient. Butter, oil, margarine, and whole milk have some, too. Just a little of this nutrient gives you a lot of energy. Too much of it can make you unhealthy by adding extra weight to your body.

You need many other nutrients as well. Some of these other nutrients help your bones and teeth. Some help your eyes, blood, or skin. Milk, fruits, and vegetables have many of these important nutrients.

One other nutrient you need is water. Most of your body is made up of water. You need water to make new cells. You also need it to stay alive. You can get some water from most foods. You should drink three to four glasses of milk, one to two glasses of juice, and several glasses of plain water each day.

Food Scientist

In the past, many people used to grow and prepare much of their food at home. Now, much food comes canned, dried, or frozen. Preparing these foods often changes their nutritional value. A *food scientist* studies the best ways to prepare, store, and cook foods so that people buy foods that are nutritious.

To be a food scientist, you need four years of college. Five years of college often is required for many jobs. To learn more about being a food scientist, write to the Institute of Food Technologists, Suite 2120, 221 North LaSalle Street, Chicago, IL 60601.

Health Career

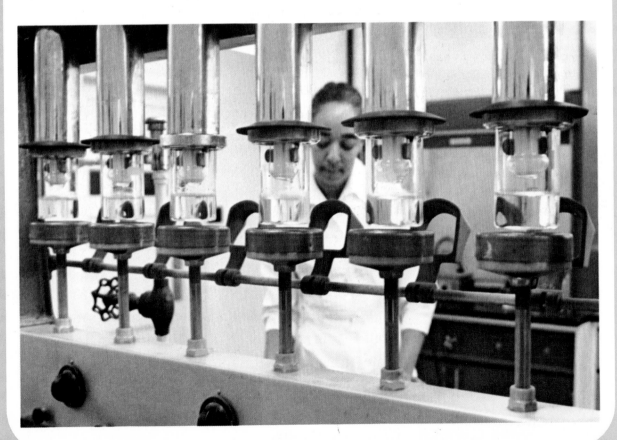

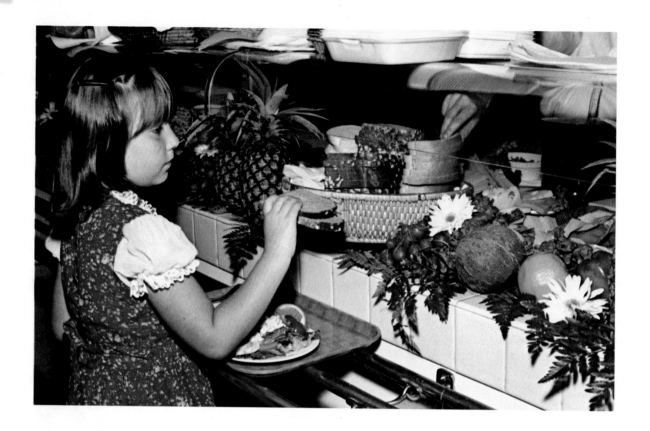

What foods can Anna choose to have with her fish that will give her the nutrients she needs?

Choosing What to Eat

Anna has decided to eat a piece of fish. But she knows that fish alone will not make a complete meal. Anna wonders what she should have with her fish.

What Anna needs are foods that will give her all the nutrients she needs. She needs something with the nutrients that fish does not have. Chicken will not do. Chicken has almost the same nutrients as fish.

Almost any green vegetable would go well with Anna's fish. Vegetables have different nutrients from fish or chicken. All foods that have almost the same nutrients belong to the same **food group.** Vegetables are in one food group. Chicken and fish are in another. All foods can be divided into four basic food groups.

Talking About Food Choices

The foods people choose to eat may depend on where they live. Why might you eat different foods than a person who lives in India? in Mexico? List at least two reasons.

Knowing about food groups can help you plan your **diet.** Your diet is the food you eat every day. A **balanced diet** includes food from each of the four basic food groups. It also includes plenty of water. A balanced diet gives you all the nutrients you need.

Wellness Tip

Snack foods sold in paper wrappers often contain a lot of added sugar or salt. For good health, eat snacks that have natural wrappers, or skins. Apples and bananas are examples.

Healthful Snacks

Eating snacks can help you have a balanced diet. Snack foods can taste good—and be good for you. Try to eat a variety of snacks from the four basic food groups. After school you could have a glass of milk and celery stuffed with peanut butter. You could eat an apple or an orange while you are waiting for the bus or watching TV. Raw vegetables, nuts, cheese, yogurt, fruit, and fruit juices are good, healthful snacks.

What healthful snacks might these children have?

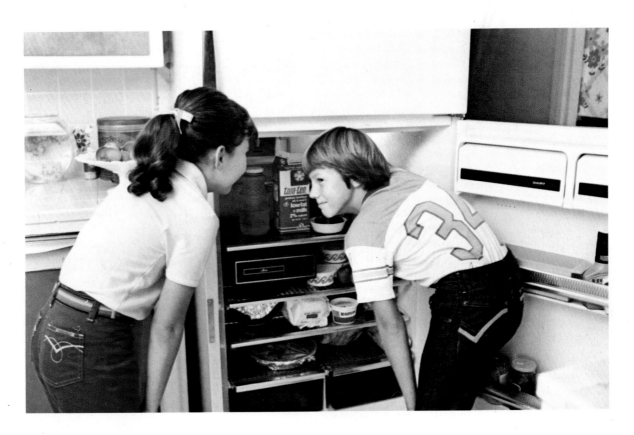

75

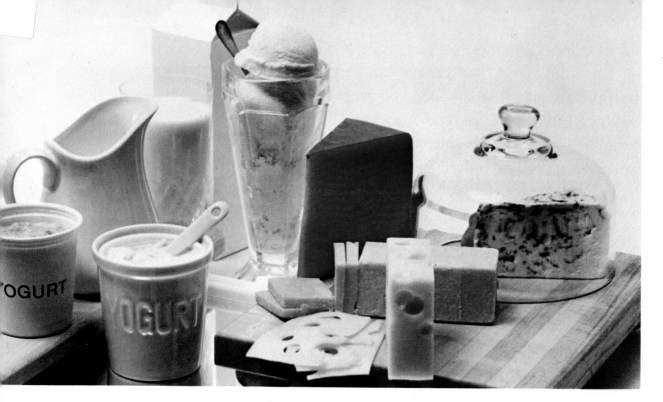

MILK GROUP

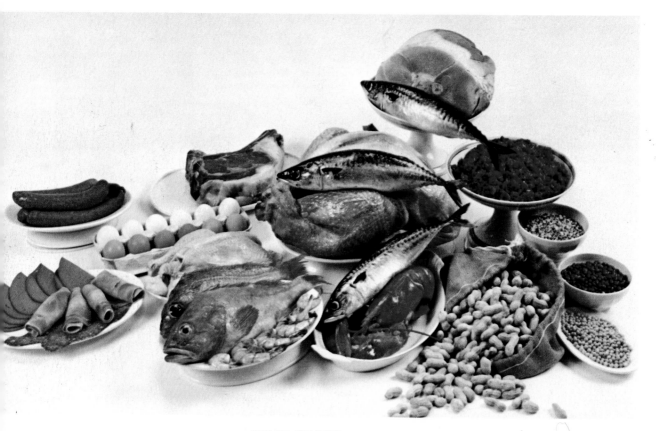

MEAT GROUP

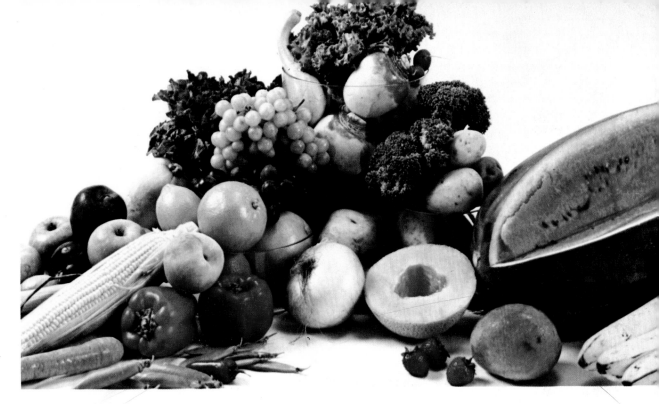

FRUIT AND VEGETABLE GROUP

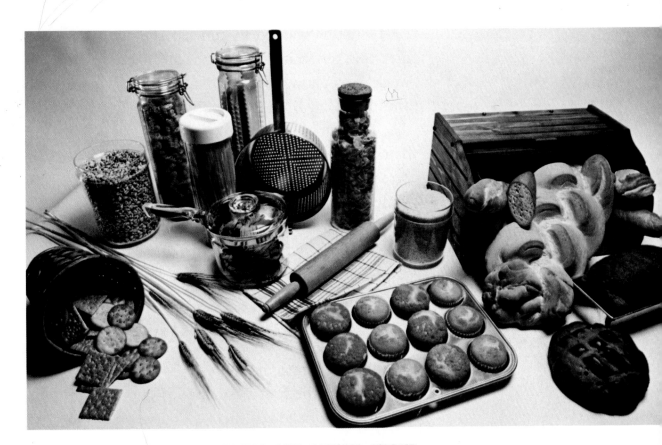

BREAD AND CEREAL GROUP

WHAT I ATE ON MONDAY

Milk Group

1 glass milk
1 glass milk
1 glass milk
4 pieces cheese

Water
3 glasses water

Bread and Cereal Group

1 slice toast
1 bun
1 dish rice
4 crackers

Meat Group

1 egg
1 hamburger
1 chicken leg

Fruit and Vegetable Group

$\frac{1}{2}$ grapefruit
1 apple
1 dish peas
1 dish green beans
1 serving tomato-green pepper sauce

How can Christina's chart help her be sure she is eating a balanced diet?

Keeping Track of What You Eat

Christina wanted to know if she ate a balanced diet. She kept track of what she ate and drank for one week. Look how Christina wrote down what she ate and drank on Monday. She wrote "hamburger" in the column for the meat group. She put the hamburger bun in the column for the bread and cereal group. Christina could see that she ate something from each food group on Monday.

Keeping track of what you eat and drink is one way to make sure you get the nutrients you need.

REVIEW IT NOW

1. What are nutrients?
2. What are the four basic food groups?
3. What is a balanced diet?
4. Why is a balanced diet important?

Making a Salad

You can plan your diet so you will get the many different nutrients your body needs. One quick way is to make a salad.

Ask a family member to help you make a salad that is rich in nutrients. Look in cookbooks for ideas, or make up your own idea for a salad. Some foods that you may want to use in your salad are spinach, mushrooms, tomatoes, avocados, cheese, raw fruits or vegetables, hard-boiled eggs, and cooked chicken. Serve the salad at one of your family's meals.

When your salad is ready to serve, you may want to choose a dressing such as oil and vinegar or yogurt and dill to go with your meal.

Working Toward Wellness

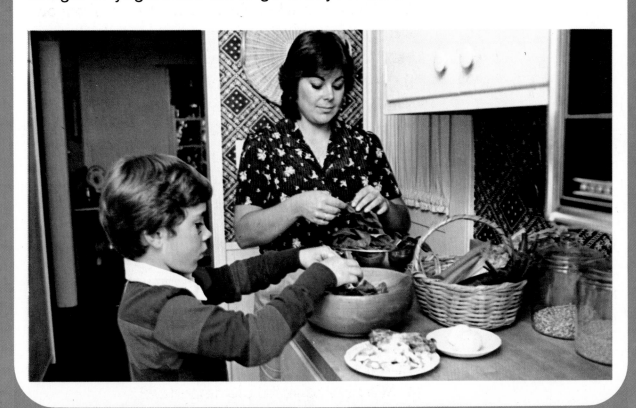

To Help You Review

Checking Your Understanding

Write the numbers from 1 to 12 on your paper. After each number, write the answer to the question. Page numbers in ( ) tell you where to look in the chapter if you need help.

1. Why are children who are the same age not all the same size and shape? (**67**)
2. Where does your body get materials to make new cells? (**70**)
3. Why do you need to eat many different kinds of food? (**72**)
4. What do the nutrients in fish, eggs, and lean meat give you? (**72**)
5. What do the nutrients found in sweet foods and fruit give you? (**72**)
6. What does the nutrient found in butter and whole milk give you? (**72**)
7. What can too much of the nutrient found in oil and margarine do to you? (**72**)
8. Why do you need water? (**72**)
9. What can a balanced diet give you? (**75**)
10. In which food group are chicken, fish, and eggs? (**76**)
11. In which food group are apples, green beans, and lettuce? (**77**)
12. How can keeping track of what you eat be helpful to you? (**78**)

Checking Your Health Vocabulary

Write the numbers from 1 to 4 on your paper. After each number, write the letter of the meaning for the word or words. Page numbers in ( ) tell you where to look in the chapter if you need help.

1. nutrients (**70**)
2. food group (**74**)
3. diet (**75**)
4. balanced diet (**75**)

a. the food you eat every day
b. parts of food that help your body grow and give you energy
c. food from each of the four basic food groups
d. foods that have almost the same nutrients

Write the numbers from 5 to 8 on your paper. After each number, write the word or words that correctly complete each sentence. Use the words from the vocabulary list above.

Margery's __(5)__ included many foods that were not nutritious. She was not getting the __(6)__ that her body needed to grow healthy and strong. So Margery decided to change her diet. She began eating foods from each __(7)__ at each meal. Margery then knew that she was eating a __(8)__ .

Practice Test

True or False?

Write the numbers from 1 to 15 on your paper. After each number, write *T* if the sentence is *true*. Write *F* if it is *false*. Rewrite each false sentence to make it true.

1. Your body grows by making bigger cells.
2. Your body is making new cells all the time.
3. Everyone grows at the same speed all the time.
4. Most girls are taller than most boys around the age of 11 or 12.
5. You use energy even to sleep.
6. Some foods have all the nutrients your body needs.
7. To stay healthy, you must eat many different kinds of food.
8. Most of your body is made up of food.
9. You do not need water to stay alive.
10. You can get some water from most foods.
11. Vegetables have the same nutrients as fish or chicken.
12. All foods are divided into three basic food groups.
13. A balanced diet includes food from each of the basic food groups.
14. A balanced diet gives you some of the nutrients you need.
15. Keeping track of what you eat and drink is one way to be sure you get the nutrients you need.

Complete the Sentence

Write the numbers from 16 to 20 on your paper. After each number, copy the sentence and fill in the missing word or words.

16. You need food for energy and _____ .
17. Your body needs many kinds of _____ .
18. Noodles and rice are in the _____ food group.
19. Knowing about food groups can help you plan your _____ .
20. A balanced diet includes food from each of the _____ basic food groups.

Learning More

For You to Do

1. Measure your height and write it down. Then weigh yourself. Write that figure down, too. Measure your height and weight once every month for six months. Keep a chart to show how much you grow during that time.

2. Cut out pictures of food from old magazines. Choose pictures that show just one kind of food, not a whole meal. Sort your pictures into the four basic food groups. Then make a poster of your pictures. The poster should show some of the different kinds of food in each food group.

3. Plan three meals your family might eat in one day. Make sure you include foods from each of the four basic food groups. Include water, juice, milk, and other healthful drinks, too.

4. Write a sentence on this subject: "Why people should eat a variety of foods." Combine your sentences with those of your classmates to make a class essay.

For You to Find Out

1. Find out what the average heights of a man and a woman were around the year 1800. What are they today? Have the average heights changed? If so, what might be a reason for such a change? Library books about growth may have the information.

2. Suppose someone did not get enough of the nutrients in milk. Find out what might happen to that person's body. What might happen if someone did not get enough of the nutrients in meat and fish? To find out, look in library books on nutrition.

For You to Read

Here are some books you can look for in your school or public library to find out more about food.

Seixas, Judith S. *Junk Food: What It Is, What It Does.* Greenwillow, 1984.

Smaridge, Norah. *What's on Your Plate?* Abingdon Press, 1982.

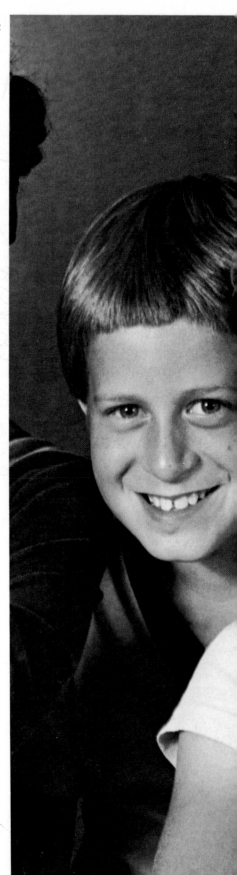

CHAPTER 4

Taking Care of Your Teeth and Gums

Your teeth and gums are very important to you. If you did not have healthy teeth and gums, you would not be able to eat many of the foods you do eat now.

All of your teeth are made of the same materials, but they have different shapes to help them do different jobs. They cut, crush, and grind the food you eat. They are the hardest parts of your body, but they still can come out or rot.

You should take care of your teeth and gums each day to keep them healthy. Healthy teeth and gums are important for your appearance. They also help you eat the foods your body needs to help you reach wellness.

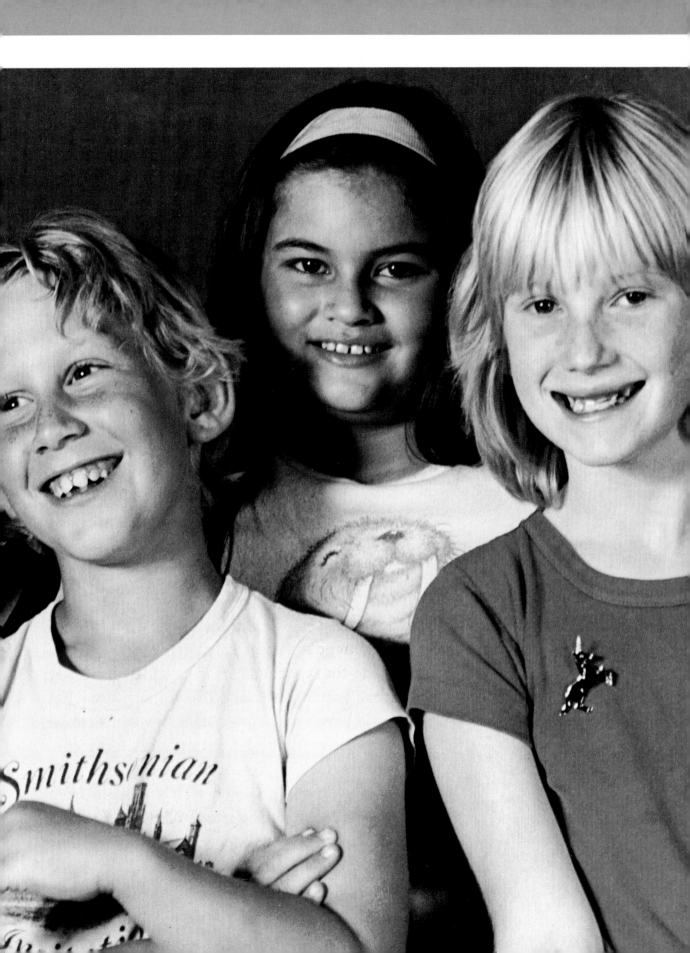

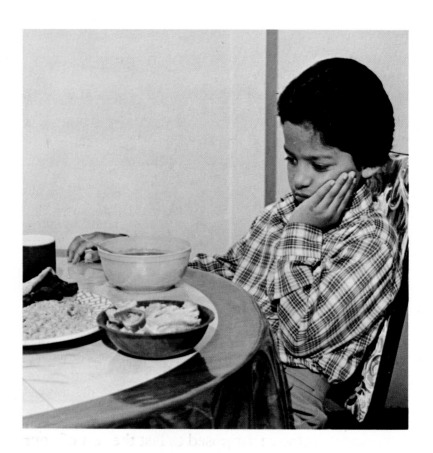

*Why must Louis eat a
nutritious soup tonight?*

YOUR TEETH

Louis sits down to dinner. He sees cornbread and pot roast on the table. But Louis has a toothache and cannot chew. So he has to make do with a nutritious soup tonight.

You need your teeth to eat many of the foods you enjoy. Chewing your food grinds it and gets it ready for your stomach. You could live without teeth, but you would have a hard time balancing your diet. All you could eat would be liquids and very soft foods.

Teeth also are important for the way you look. Have you ever seen a person with a missing front tooth? Usually the person tries to hide it or smiles differently. The way your teeth look can change the way you feel about yourself.

Using Teeth in Talking

Your teeth are important for the way you talk. Say the word *teeth.* Your tongue and teeth help you make the sounds for *t* and *th.* Now say the word *five.* Your lips and teeth help you make the sounds *f* and *v.* There are many words you cannot say without using your teeth.

Your First Set of Teeth

Two sets of teeth will grow in your mouth. Your first set of teeth began growing in when you were about six months old. These were your baby teeth, or **primary teeth.** You had only 20 of these teeth. You have probably lost some of them already. You started losing your primary teeth when you were about six years old. You probably will lose the last one when you are 12 or 13.

Your Second Set of Teeth

As your first teeth are lost, your second set grows in. These are your adult teeth, or **permanent teeth.** This set has 32 teeth. Your first permanent tooth probably grew in a year or two ago. You should have your full set of permanent teeth by your late teens. Permanent teeth are supposed to last the rest of your life. If you lose one of them, your body cannot grow another. You may need a false tooth.

Deciding About Baby Teeth

Eddy was playing tag with his older brother. Eddy fell. He knocked out one of his front teeth. "Don't worry," Eddy's brother said. "It's just one of your baby teeth. Your baby teeth are not very important." Was Eddy's brother right? Why or why not?

How many primary teeth are shown here? How many permanent teeth are shown?

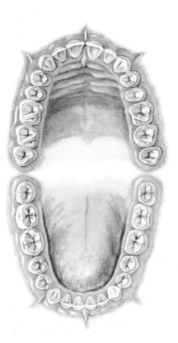

Different Kinds of Teeth

You have four kinds of teeth. Each kind has a different shape and works in a different way. You need all four kinds to chew properly.

Teeth for Cutting and Tearing

Fritz is eating a hamburger. To take a bite, he uses teeth in the front of his mouth. These teeth have sharp edges and flat tops. They are called **incisors.** You have eight incisors. Four of them are in your upper jaw. Four more are in your lower jaw. The upper and lower incisors work together, like scissor blades. You use your incisors mainly to cut your food.

The teeth on either side of the incisors tear your food. These teeth come to a point at the top. They are called **cuspids.** You have two cuspids in your upper jaw and two in your lower jaw.

What teeth is Fritz using to take the first bite of his hamburger?

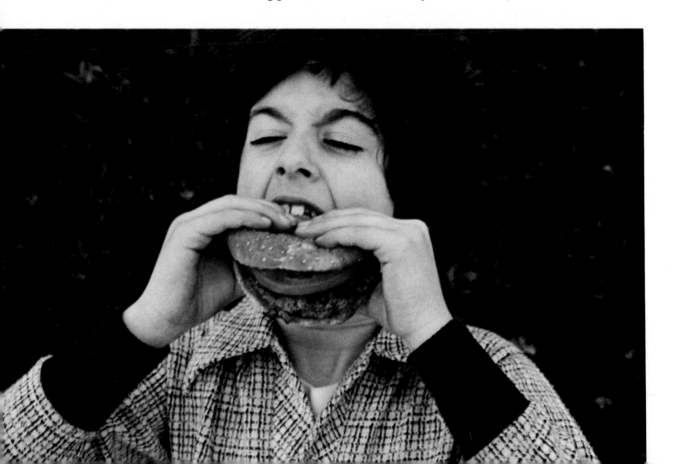

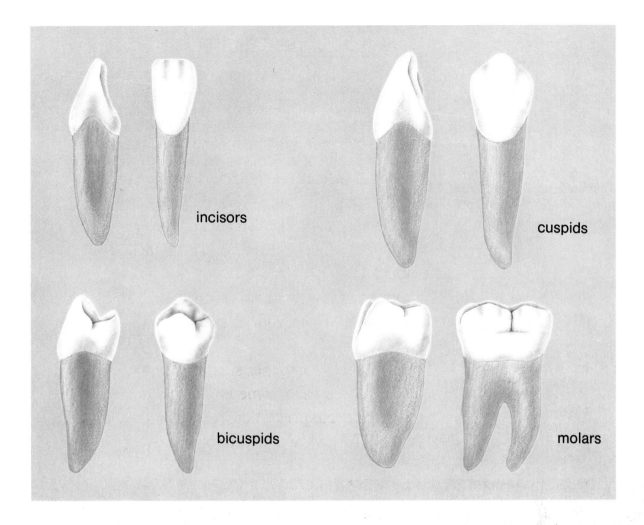

incisors

cuspids

bicuspids

molars

Teeth for Grinding and Crushing

When Fritz chews his bite of hamburger, the food moves to his back teeth. These teeth grind and crush the food into a thick liquid.

Some of the back teeth have two points. They are called **bicuspids.** You may not have any bicuspids yet. Other teeth do their job for now. In a few years you probably will have eight bicuspids.

Your **molars** are the wide teeth in the very back of your mouth. Each molar has a broad top with several points. When you chew, the upper and lower molars press against each other. They crush and grind the food between them.

Look at the shape of each tooth. How might each shape help cut, tear, or grind and crush food?

Six-year Molars

Six-year molars are important. They must do the heavy work of chewing while your primary teeth are being replaced by permanent teeth.

Your Wisdom Teeth

The four molars at the very back of your mouth are your **wisdom teeth.** If all your permanent teeth grow in, you will have two wisdom teeth on top and two on bottom. Your wisdom teeth will not grow in until you reach your late teens or early twenties. Some people's wisdom teeth never grow in. People without wisdom teeth have no problems talking or chewing their food.

Which teeth cut your food? Which tear your food? Which grind and crush your food?

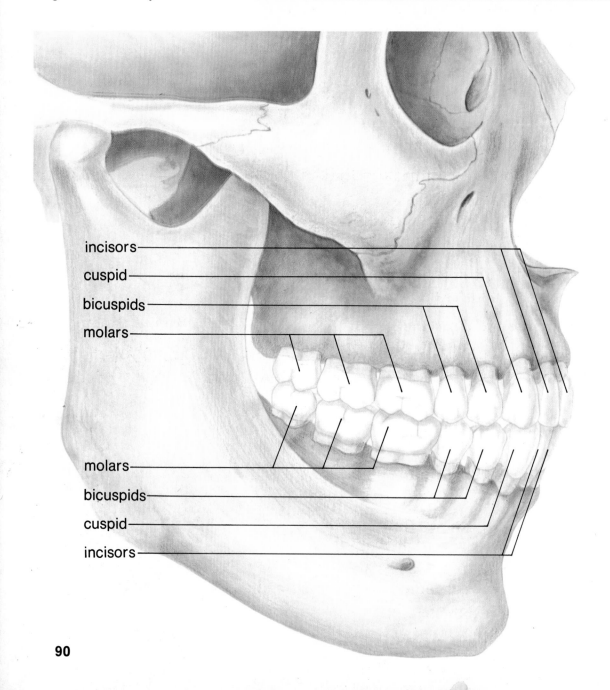

incisors
cuspid
bicuspids
molars

molars
bicuspids
cuspid
incisors

Fixing a Tooth with Plastic

A chipped or broken tooth can ruin a nice smile and cause more serious dental problems. What can be done to make the tooth look like it did before it was damaged?

Dentists can use different ways to repair a damaged front tooth. One of these ways is called *bonding.* Bonding is a way to repair a tooth by using a substance called *resin.* Resin is a sticky, liquid plastic.

Dentists can often bond a tooth without drilling into the tooth. The enamel around the damaged area of the tooth is painted with a special liquid. This liquid makes the enamel rough, like sandpaper. Resin is then painted in layers onto the rough surface until it fills in the damaged area. After the resin gets hard, the dentist polishes the resin to make it smooth. The tooth now looks like it did before it was damaged.

Health Today

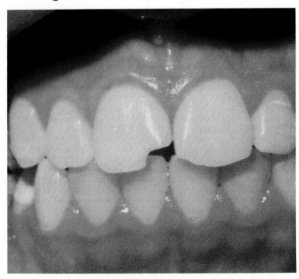
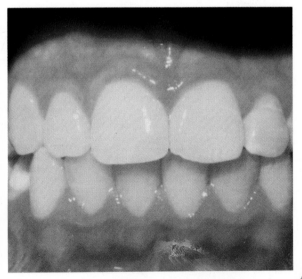

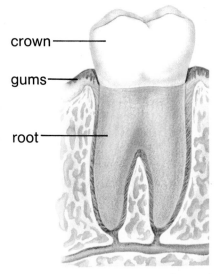

crown——

gums——

root——

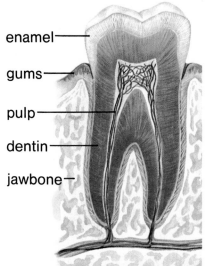

enamel——

gums——

pulp——

dentin——

jawbone——

What part of the tooth do you see when you look into the mirror?

What a Tooth Is Like

Smile into a mirror and look at one of your teeth. You are looking at only part of the tooth. The part you can see is called the **crown.** Almost half of the tooth is hidden by your **gums.** Your gums are the pink tissue around your teeth. The hidden part of the tooth is called the **root.** The roots of your teeth go through your gums and into your jawbone.

A tooth has many layers. Each layer is different. The picture shows the different parts of the tooth.

The **enamel** is the outer layer. It makes a thin, hard shell around the tooth. Enamel is even harder than bone. It protects your tooth. **Dentin** is a thick layer under the enamel. Dentin is hard, too. But it is not as hard as enamel.

Dentin and enamel are made by the living part of the tooth. This part is the **pulp.** It is in a hollow space in the very middle of the tooth. The pulp is soft tissue with nerves and blood vessels. The pulp works to keep the rest of the tooth healthy.

REVIEW IT NOW

1. What are primary teeth?
2. What is your second set of teeth called?
3. What are the four kinds of teeth that you have?
4. What are the names of three layers of the tooth?

Ann Kristovich

Dr. Ann Kristovich is an oral surgeon. Oral surgeons are dentists who are trained to perform special kinds of operations. They remove wisdom teeth, fix broken jaws, and treat diseases of the mouth.

Ann performs some operations in her office. Other operations need to be done in the hospital. For example, Ann went to the hospital to treat a young person who had fallen off his bicycle. He had broken his jaw. She wired his teeth together to give the jaw a chance to heal.

Dr. Kristovich likes to work with people. She also likes to solve difficult problems. Oral surgery gives her a chance to do both.

Focus On

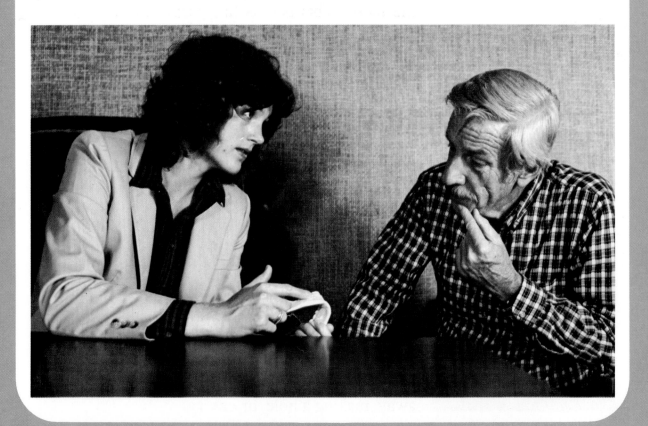

93

This is what plaque looks like when seen through a microscope.

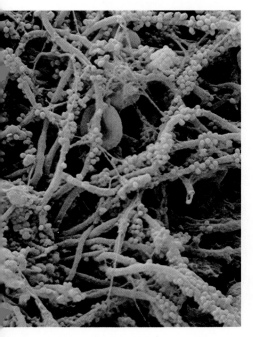

TAKING CARE OF YOUR TEETH

Your teeth can rot, or **decay,** if you do not take good care of them. Decayed teeth look bad. They can cause you a lot of pain, too. You may even lose a tooth that is decayed. Taking good care of your teeth can help prevent decay.

You cannot chew or talk as well as you should if you are missing any of your teeth. Even if you lose only one tooth, it can make a difference. If you lose a permanent tooth, you cannot grow another one to replace it. You may have to get a false tooth.

You should take good care of your primary teeth, too. They are important even though permanent teeth will replace them. If you let your primary teeth decay, they may be lost too soon. The shape of your mouth could change. This could change how your permanent teeth grow in. Your permanent teeth might grow in crooked. Or your top and bottom teeth might not meet as they should. You would probably find it difficult to chew.

How Tooth Decay Happens

After you eat, bits of food often stay on your teeth. Food and microbes stick together. They form a clear, gooey substance called **plaque.**

Certain microbes live in plaque. They live on sugar from the food you eat. They make **acids.** The acids are sour substances that are very strong. They can break down tooth enamel. The enamel wears away, making a hole, or **cavity.**

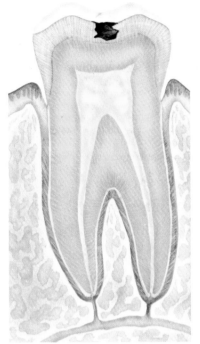 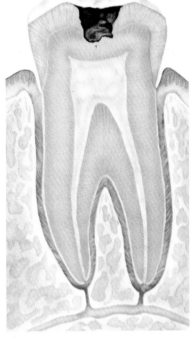 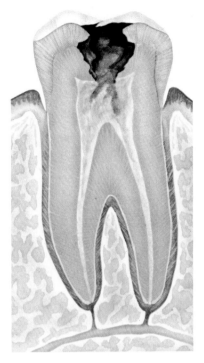

Unless the cavity is filled, it gets bigger. It goes into the dentin. Finally it reaches the pulp. Acids and microbes may destroy the pulp and kill the tooth.

What happens to a tooth if a cavity is not filled?

How Gum Damage Happens

Plaque can harm your gums, too. If plaque stays on your teeth too long, it forms **calculus** (tartar). Calculus is a hard, yellow substance. It forms between the gums and teeth and makes a space between them. Microbes grow in this space and harm the gums.

When gums are damaged, they look red instead of pink. They bleed easily when you brush your teeth. They may be too soft to hold your teeth in place. In some cases, the jawbone holding the teeth also becomes diseased. Then the teeth become loose and may even come out.

Talking About Teeth

With a friend, talk about how each of the things below could damage teeth or gums:
- chewing on a pen or pencil
- chewing gum
- playing a rough sport such as football

95

Cleaning Your Teeth and Gums

Plaque causes problems for both your gums and your teeth. But you can clean the plaque off your teeth. Then you can prevent most gum and tooth problems.

These pictures show Rick and Tina cleaning their teeth. Rick is using a toothbrush. Tina has brushed her teeth already. Now she is using **dental floss.** Dental floss is a special kind of white string. Using it removes plaque and food from between your teeth and cleans along your gumline. Dental floss cleans spots that a toothbrush cannot reach.

Your dentist or **dental hygienist** can show you the best ways to brush and floss. A dental hygienist cleans your teeth and tells you how to take care of them. You should brush your teeth after every meal. If you cannot brush after a meal, rinse your mouth with water. Rinsing removes some bits of food. You should floss your teeth once a day, at bedtime.

Why is it important to use dental floss after brushing your teeth?

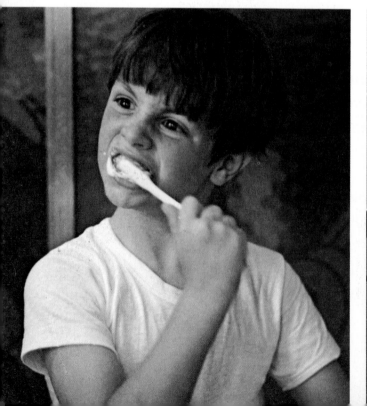

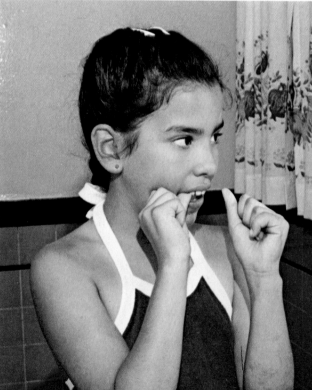

Dental Hygienist

A person who helps your dentist take care of your teeth is a *dental hygienist*. A dental hygienist examines, cleans, and polishes teeth. The hygienist also teaches people the proper ways to care for their teeth and gums.

Most dental hygienists work in dentists' offices. Others work in schools, health clinics, hospitals, and retirement homes.

A person who wants to become a dental hygienist must complete a two-year program in dental hygiene. A state license also is required. To learn more about being a dental hygienist, write to the American Dental Hygienists' Association, 444 North Michigan Avenue, Chicago, IL 60611.

Health Career

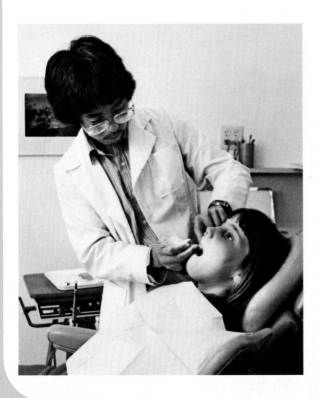

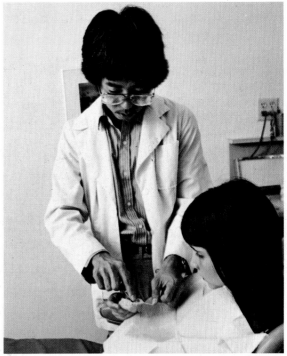

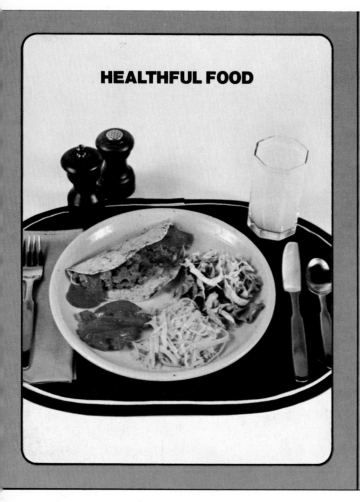

HEALTHFUL FOOD

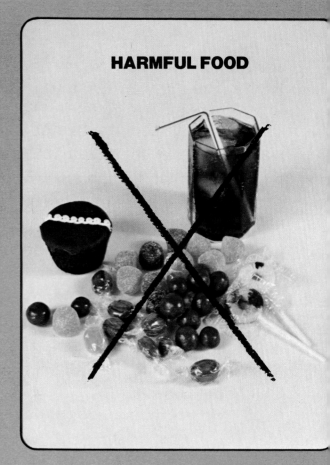

HARMFUL FOOD

How can eating healthful foods help your teeth? How can eating foods with sugar harm your teeth?

Eating Healthful Foods

You can help your teeth stay healthy by making them strong. You can make them strong by eating foods that have enough of the nutrients your teeth need. Milk and other foods in the milk group help build strong teeth.

Some foods can harm your teeth. Sugar probably is the most harmful food for teeth. The microbes that cause tooth decay live on sugar. You should not eat too many foods that contain a lot of sugar. Also, you should brush your teeth or rinse your mouth with water right after eating any sweet food. This helps protect your teeth from cavities.

Seeing Your Dentist

Even when you take proper care of your teeth, you may still get a cavity sometimes. If you do not have a cavity fixed right away, it grows large. Then it can cause a bad toothache. But if you visit your dentist often, you may never get a toothache. Your dentist can fill a cavity when it is small. Then the cavity never becomes large.

Your dentist may have a dental hygienist to clean your teeth and tell you how to care for them. The hygienist can clean your teeth better than you can by using special tools.

Louis is visiting his dentist to have a cavity filled. How can visiting a dentist often help prevent cavities?

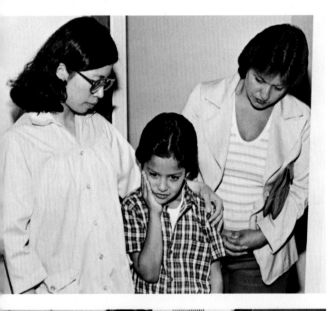

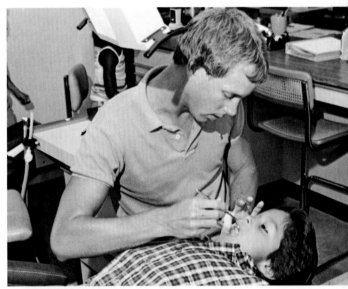

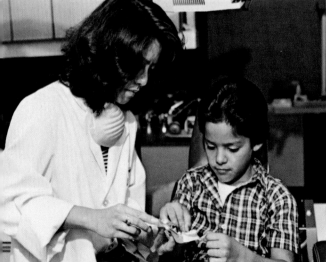

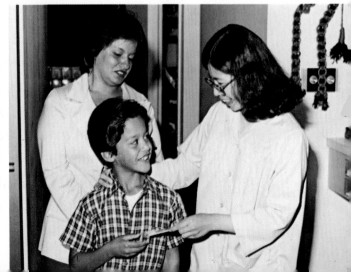

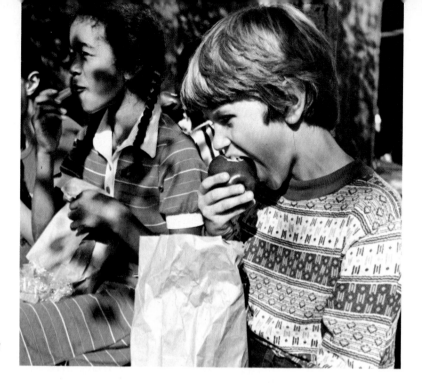

How can strong teeth help you stay healthy?

Talking About Healthy Teeth

With a friend or a classmate talk about what makes healthy teeth. How can a person tell if his or her teeth are healthy?

Many people visit a dentist at least once a year. At your age it might be wise to visit one every six months. That is because you are losing one set of teeth and growing another set.

Taking care of your teeth is important for your health. Healthy teeth make you look and feel better. They help you enjoy many kinds of food so that you can eat what you need for growth. If you take proper care of your teeth now, they should last you the rest of your life.

REVIEW IT NOW

1. What happens if a permanent tooth is lost?
2. What is plaque?
3. What is a cavity?
4. What is dental floss used for?
5. What foods help build strong teeth?
6. What foods can harm your teeth?

Keeping a Teeth-care Chart

Are you taking good care of your teeth? You can check your teeth-care habits by keeping a chart for one week. You may want to encourage a family member to keep one, too.

Make a chart like the one in the picture. Place it near where you keep your toothbrush. At the end of each day, fill in your chart. How did you clean your teeth after each meal? Write "b" for brush, "f" for floss, or "r" for rinse.

At the end of the week, look over your chart. Are there any blank spaces? Your chart should help you see how you can improve your teeth-care habits.

Working Toward Wellness

	Mon.	Tues.	Wed.	Thurs.	Fri.	Sat.	Sun.
Breakfast	b		b	b	b	b	b
	f		f	f		f	f
	r	r		r	r	r	r
Lunch		b	b		b	b	b
	r	r	r	r	r	r	r
Dinner	b	b	b	b	b	b	b
	f	f	f	f	f	f	f
	r	r	r	r	r	r	r

To Help You Review

Checking Your Understanding

Write the numbers from 1 to 15 on your paper. After each number, write the answer to the question. Page numbers in ( ) tell you where to look in the chapter if you need help.

1. What are two reasons your teeth are important? **(86)**
2. Why do you need four kinds of teeth? **(88)**
3. What do incisors do when you eat? **(88)**
4. What do cuspids do when you eat? **(88)**
5. Which teeth grind and crush your food? **(89)**
6. What are the four molars at the very back of your mouth called? **(90)**
7. What are the two hard layers of your tooth called? **(92)**
8. What is the living part of a tooth? **(92)**
9. What can taking good care of your teeth help prevent? **(94)**
10. What may happen if your primary teeth are lost too soon? **(94)**
11. How do the microbes that live in plaque start a cavity? **(94)**
12. What happens if a cavity is not filled? **(95)**
13. How can calculus harm your gums? **(95)**
14. How do damaged gums look? **(95)**
15. How can using dental floss help your teeth? **(96)**

Checking Your Health Vocabulary

Write the numbers from 1 to 6 on your paper. After each number, write the letter of the meaning for the word or words. Page numbers in ( ) tell you where to look in the chapter if you need help.

1. crown (**92**)
2. gums (**92**)
3. root (**92**)
4. enamel (**92**)
5. dentin (**92**)
6. pulp (**92**)

a. the hidden part of a tooth
b. soft tissue with nerves and blood inside a tooth
c. the part of the tooth you can see
d. a thick layer under the enamel
e. the thin, hard outer layer of a tooth
f. the pink tissue around your teeth

Write the numbers from 7 to 15 on your paper. Then write a sentence that explains the meaning of each word or words. Page numbers in ( ) tell you where to look in the chapter if you need help.

7. primary teeth (**87**)
8. permanent teeth (**87**)
9. decay (**94**)
10. plaque (**94**)
11. acids (**94**)
12. cavity (**94**)
13. calculus (**95**)
14. dental floss (**96**)
15. dental hygienist (**96**)

Practice Test

True or False?

Write the numbers from 1 to 15 on your paper. After each number, write *T* if the sentence is *true*. Write *F* if it is *false*. Rewrite each false sentence to make it true.

1. You need your teeth to eat many of the foods you enjoy.
2. The way your teeth look can change the way you feel about yourself.
3. Two sets of teeth will grow in your mouth.
4. Your permanent teeth began growing in when you were about six months old.
5. If you lose a permanent tooth, your body grows another to take its place.
6. You have four incisors.
7. Some people's wisdom teeth never grow in.
8. A tooth's enamel is harder than bone.
9. Dentin and enamel are made by the gums.
10. If you lose your primary teeth too soon, it could change how your permanent teeth grow in.
11. If a cavity is not filled, it may kill the tooth.
12. If you brush every day, you do not need to use dental floss.
13. Foods in the milk group help build strong teeth.
14. The microbes that cause tooth decay live on milk.
15. It is a good idea to see a dentist once every two years.

Complete the Sentence

Write the numbers from 16 to 20 on your paper. After each number, copy the sentence and fill in the missing word or words.

16. A full set of _____ teeth has 20 teeth.
17. You need _____ different kinds of teeth to chew properly.
18. The part of a tooth you can see is called the _____ .
19. The roots of your teeth go through your _____ .
20. _____ probably is the most harmful food for teeth.

Learning More

For You to Do

1. Take a bite of an apple. Which teeth did you use? Chew the piece of apple. Notice how it moved to your back teeth. Which teeth did you use to chew and crush the piece of food?

2. Prepare a report for your class about *fluoride* and the way it may help your teeth. Look in library books about teeth or ask your dentist for information about fluoride.

For You to Find Out

1. Decayed permanent teeth are often pulled and replaced with false teeth. But there is a way to save some decayed teeth. Ask your dentist or read library books to find out about *root canal* operations and how root canal operations can help save decayed teeth.

2. Dentists who straighten people's teeth are called *orthodontists*. How does an orthodontist straighten teeth? Why are straight teeth important for health? Talk with an orthodontist or your dentist to find out.

3. A tooth can become cracked or chipped. This damages the enamel and dentin. It can cause damage to the rest of the tooth, too. Find out how dentists repair cracked or chipped teeth to protect them from further damage. Ask your dentist or look in library books about teeth.

For You to Read

Here are some books you can look for in your school or public library to find out more about your teeth.

Betancourt, Jeanne. *Smile! How to Cope with Braces*. Knopf, 1982.

Krementz, Jill. *Taryn Goes to the Dentist*. Crown Publishers, 1986.

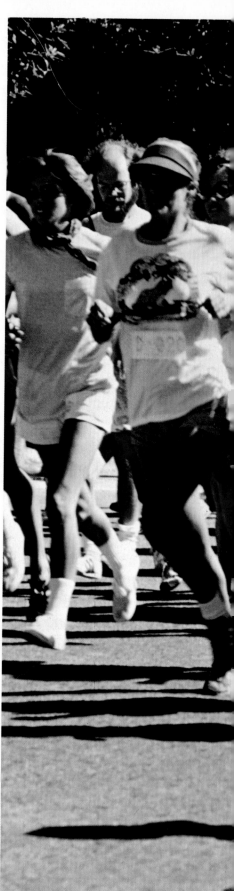

CHAPTER 5

Exercise, Rest, and Sleep

Think about the things you like to do outdoors. Do you like to run? Perhaps you like to swim, skate, or play ball with friends.

These activities can be fun. They can also help you reach and keep up your wellness. These activities and others like them make your muscles, heart, and lungs work fast and hard. This makes your whole body stronger.

No matter how strong you are, you get tired. You need to rest and sleep every day. Your body stores its energy while you rest and sleep. After sleeping or resting, you have the energy you need again.

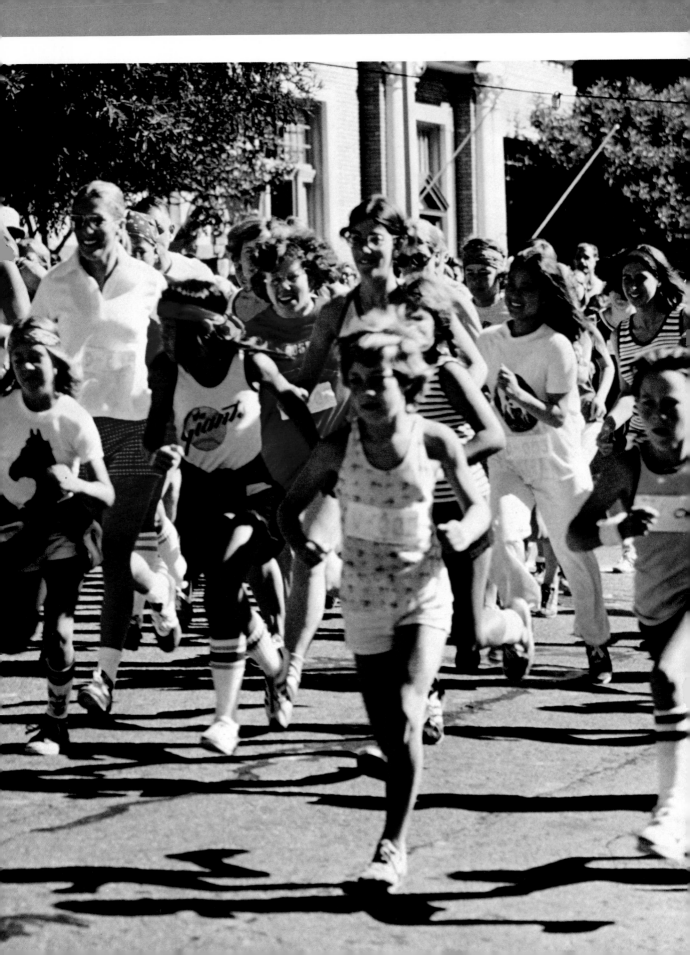

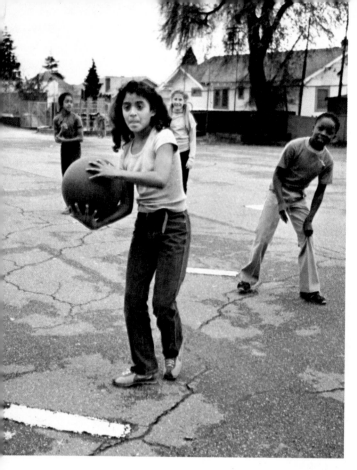

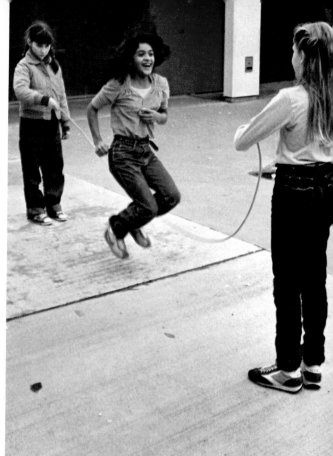

How is Martha's body getting exercise?

EXERCISING TO LOOK AND FEEL YOUR BEST

Martha usually has a very active day. She walks to school. She plays kickball at recess. After school, she jumps rope with her friends. All of these activities make Martha's body work hard. Any activity that makes your body work hard is **exercise.**

Regular exercise helps your body work at its best. It makes your heart and other muscles strong. It makes your lungs able to hold more air. It makes your blood move quickly to all of the cells in your body. Then your blood can take nutrients and oxygen to your cells quickly. It can quickly carry away your cells' wastes, too. This will help all of your cells, tissues, and organs work at their best.

Exercise and Fitness

Regular exercise helps your body keep physically fit. When you are physically fit, all of the parts of your body can work at their best. Your body is healthy. You look and feel healthy, too.

Exercising to Use Food

You need to eat a balanced diet to have a healthy body. You also need to exercise. Exercise helps your body turn the nutrients from food into energy. If you do not get enough exercise, your body does not use up food. Instead of giving you energy, some food turns to fat. And you can become tired easily.

Each day Kevin eats the food his body needs. Food gives his body energy to work and play.

Kevin also exercises every day. He makes his body work hard. Some days he runs races with his friends. Some days he jumps rope. He plays soccer at school. He swims and rides his bicycle.

Kevin likes to exercise. It is fun for him and it makes his body feel good. It also makes his body strong and healthy.

When Kevin exercises, he uses the energy from food. He can work and play hard for a long time before becoming tired.

Keeping Track of Your Exercise

For one week, keep track of all the exercise you get. Maybe you walk to school or the store. Maybe you ride a bike. Maybe you play active games. Write down all the kinds of exercise you get each day.

From what does Kevin's body get the extra energy it needs during exercise?

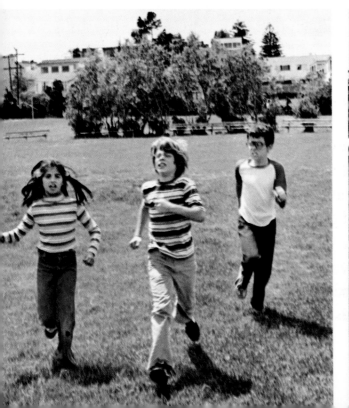
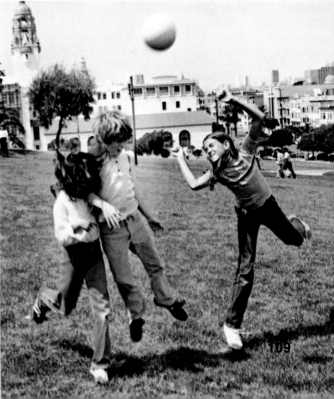

109

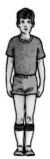

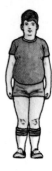

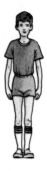

Food, Exercise, and Your Weight

The amount of food you eat and the amount of exercise you get should be in balance. If they are in balance, your weight will stay the same.

But, if you eat more food than your body can use through exercise, or if you do not exercise to use the food you eat, you will gain weight.

If you do not eat enough food for your body to use, your body will use some of its stored food. You will lose weight.

If you want to change your weight, you can change the amount of food you eat or the amount of exercise you get. You should see a doctor before you change either.

If the amount of food you eat and the amount of exercise you get are in balance, what will happen to your weight?

Exercising Your Muscles

Regular exercise helps your muscles in three ways. It makes them stronger. It makes them able to work longer without becoming tired. And it makes them able to stretch easily.

Some exercises help your muscles in all three ways. Other exercises help them in only one or two ways. You need to do different kinds of exercises to help your muscles in all three ways.

110

Kathy, Carlos, and Betty get plenty of exercise each day. They know that regular exercise helps their muscles work well.

Carlos is doing sit-ups. He does some every day. At first he could do only a few. But each day he can do one or two more. Exercising regularly is helping his muscles become strong.

Six weeks ago Betty became tired after swimming three lengths of the pool. Now she can swim ten lengths. Regular exercise has helped her muscles be able to work a long time without tiring.

When Kathy started learning to dance, she found it difficult to bend and stretch. Her body felt sore. Now she can move smoothly without feeling sore. Exercising regularly has helped her muscles. She can bend and stretch more easily.

Talking About a World Without Exercise

Imagine a future world in which no one exercises. Machines do everything for people. How might this affect people's muscles? What might a person who lives in such a world look like?

How has regular exercise helped Carlos's muscles? How has regular exercise helped Kathy's muscles?

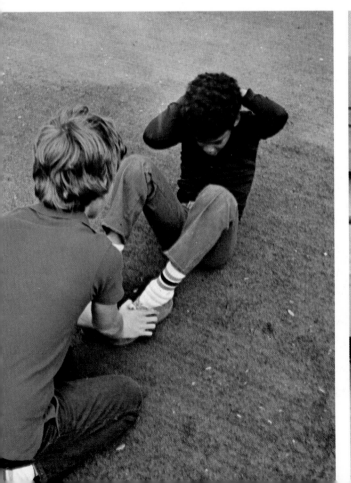

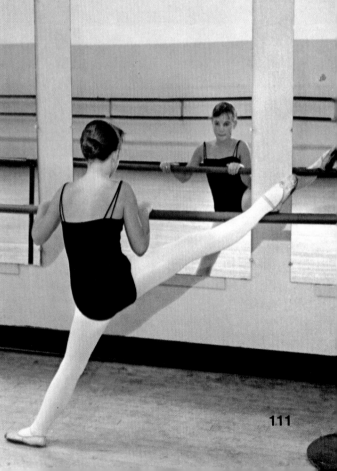

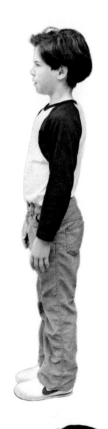

Exercising for Good Posture

The way you hold your body is called your **posture.** When you have good posture, your body systems can do the work they are supposed to do. Good posture helps your bones grow properly. It gives the organs inside your body room to work. Your lungs can get plenty of air. The parts of your digestive system have room to work, too.

You need strong muscles to have good posture. Strong muscles help hold your spine straight. They help your feet and legs support your weight.

Weak muscles can cause poor posture. They can get tired, stiff, and sore. They can make parts of your body ache. They can cause you to slump your shoulders or your back. Then your muscles may hurt even more.

Getting regular exercise keeps your muscles strong and helps you have good posture. That makes you look better. It also helps your body work at its best.

REVIEW IT NOW

1. What is exercise?
2. In what three ways can regular exercise help your muscles?
3. What is posture?
4. In what ways does good posture help your body?
5. How does regular exercise help give you good posture?

In what way can regular exercise help your posture?

Pat Fukahara

Pat Fukahara enjoys working with students. She teaches at a high school in Los Angeles. She coaches a basketball team for the Special Olympics, too.

The Special Olympics gives handicapped people experience in sports. The experience makes them feel good about themselves. Success in the Special Olympics means that every player has tried his or her best. Winning is not important. As a coach, Pat Fukahara sees to it that every player succeeds. She gives support and encouragement to her team members. Pat knows that success on the basketball court can help each person's self-esteem.

Focus On

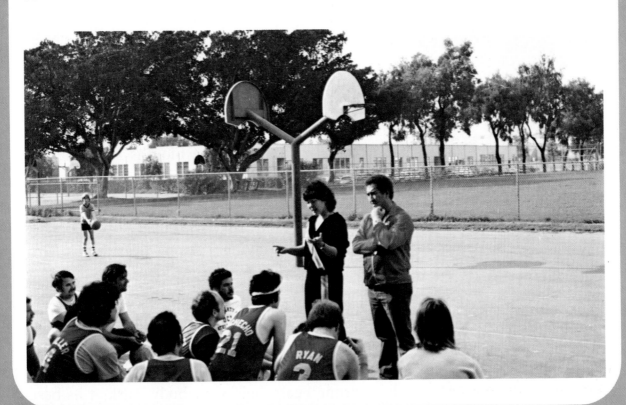

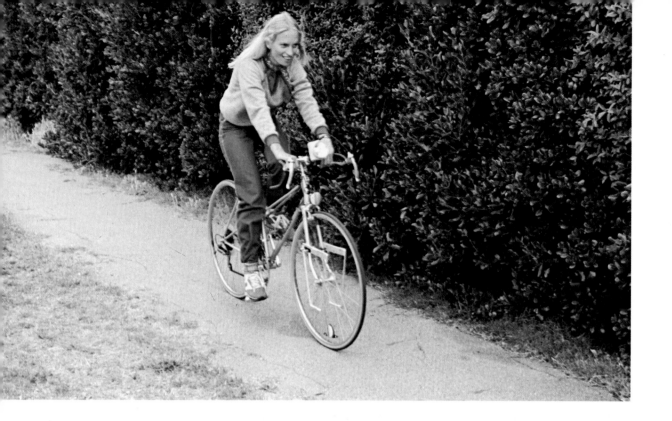

How has bicycling regularly helped Mrs. Kaminsky's muscles?

EXERCISING FOR YOUR HEART AND LUNGS

Mrs. Kaminsky is riding her bicycle. She started riding three months ago. At first she could ride only a few miles before she became tired. Now she can ride 10 miles (16 km).

Bicycling has given Mrs. Kaminsky more strength than she had three months ago. She can work longer without feeling tired.

Bicycling has made Mrs. Kaminsky's muscles strong. It has made her heart strong, too. The heart is made of muscle. Having a strong heart helps Mrs. Kaminsky keep healthy.

Exercising makes your heart beat fast. It makes you breathe fast, too. When you breathe fast, your lungs have to work hard. If your lungs work hard every day, they can hold more air. Healthy lungs, like a strong heart, help your body work at its best.

Getting Oxygen

Brenda is running in a race. She is running as fast as she can. Her muscles are using a lot of energy.

Brenda needs extra energy to run the race. Her muscles get energy from the nutrients in food stored in her body. Brenda helps her body get the energy it needs. She breathes fast and hard. She breathes in extra oxygen. The oxygen helps Brenda get the stored nutrients to her muscles. Now Brenda can get the energy she needs.

When the race is over, Brenda will feel out of breath. Her body will have worked hard during the race. She will be breathing fast. But soon after the race, Brenda's body will be doing less work. She will need less oxygen. She will not need to breathe fast any longer.

How is Brenda getting stored nutrients to her muscles as she runs the race?

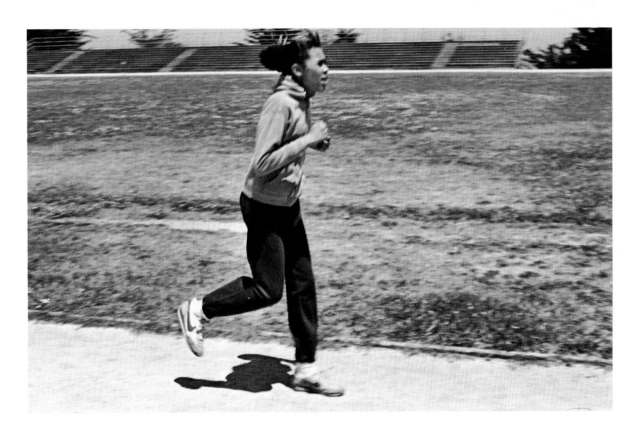

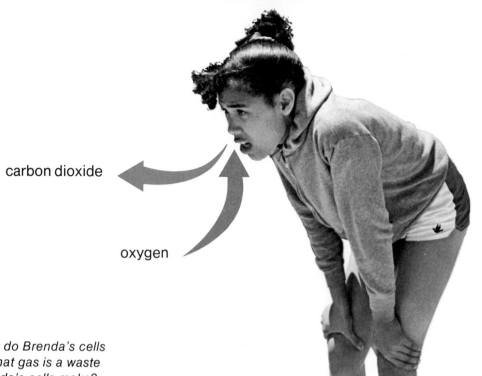

carbon dioxide

oxygen

What gas do Brenda's cells need? What gas is a waste that Brenda's cells make?

Getting Rid of Wastes

When Brenda exercises by running, her cells quickly use nutrients in food for energy. As cells use these nutrients, they make wastes. One waste is carbon dioxide. Another waste is water.

Brenda's blood carries carbon dioxide and water to her lungs. Carbon dioxide leaves her body when she breathes out. A small amount of water leaves her body this way, too.

When you exercise, your lungs work hard. You take in more oxygen than usual. More wastes leave your body.

Moving Your Blood Quickly

When Brenda is racing, her blood moves quickly throughout her body. It is carrying oxygen to her cells and carrying away wastes. Her heart works hard to pump blood around her body.

About Your Heart

Your heart beats slowly when you are asleep. It beats fast when you are very active, or when you are angry or afraid.

When you exercise, your heart beats faster than when you sit still. It pumps more blood to carry extra oxygen to your muscles. Your muscles need extra oxygen when they work hard. By pumping more blood, your heart also helps your cells get rid of the extra wastes they are making.

Making Your Heart Stronger

Each time your heart beats, it pushes blood through your arteries. The push of blood through your arteries with each heartbeat is your **pulse.**

Regular exercise makes your heart muscle stronger. Your heart beats more slowly and pumps more blood each time it beats.

Before Mr. Swanson began playing tennis regularly, he counted his pulse while he was sitting quietly. He found that his heart beat 70 times a minute. After three months of regular exercise, Mr. Swanson's heart beats only 60 times a minute when he is sitting still. Exercising has made Mr. Swanson's heart stronger.

Taking Your Pulse

The picture at the bottom of the page shows how to take a pulse. Take your pulse. Then run in place for one minute. Now take your pulse again. How has it changed? Why has it changed?

Mr. Swanson is taking his pulse. To take your pulse, press your index finger and middle finger on the side of your neck where you feel a heartbeat. Count the number of heartbeats you feel in one minute. The number of heartbeats per minute is your pulse.

117

How might roller-skating help your heart? How might bicycling help your lungs?

Exercises That Help Your Heart and Lungs

You can make your lungs take in more oxygen by exercising. You can also make your heart stronger by exercising. Then your blood will be able to carry oxygen to your cells more quickly. Your whole body will work better.

Exercise that makes your heart beat fast helps your heart the most. Running slowly and steadily helps your heart. Swimming, roller-skating, and playing games like soccer also help your heart.

Exercise that makes you breathe hard helps your lungs the most. For example, riding a bicycle or running races with a friend after school are exercises that help your lungs.

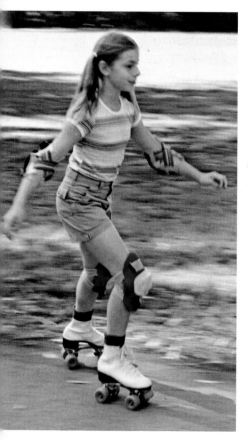

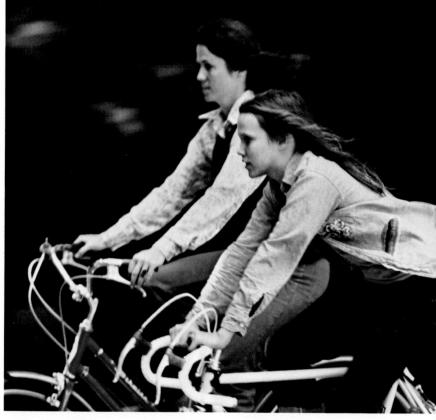

Bob decided to exercise to help both his heart and his lungs. He started jumping rope. Jumping rope made his heart beat fast. It made him breathe hard, too.

Bob kept track of how much exercise he got each day. The week he started exercising, he jumped rope without resting for three minutes each day. The second week he raised the time to five minutes each day. He raised the time just a little each week. After eight weeks, Bob was jumping rope fast for ten minutes every day. Then he cut back to jumping five times a week.

By getting regular exercise, Bob is making his heart and lungs work at their best. Making your heart and lungs work well when you are young can help you all your life. If you keep your heart and lungs working well, you will be healthy for many years.

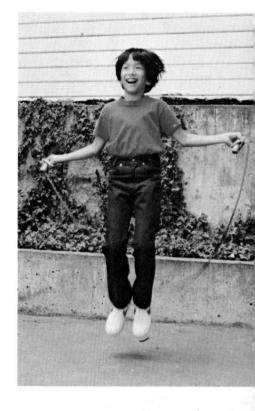

How can jumping rope regularly help Bob's heart?

REVIEW IT NOW

1. What happens to your lungs if they work hard every day?
2. Why does your heart beat faster when you are exercising than when you are resting?
3. What is your pulse?
4. What does regular exercise do for your heart?
5. To help your lungs, what should exercising make you do?

Physical Education Teacher

Health Career

A person who enjoys exercise, active games, and working with students may want to become a *physical education teacher*. The physical education teacher knows the kinds of exercise and activities that are good for growing bodies. With the physical education teacher's guidance, students can exercise their bodies in safe and healthful ways.

To be a physical education teacher, you need four years of college. Each state also has its own requirements for its teachers. To learn more about being a physical education teacher, write to the American Federation of Teachers, 555 New Jersey Avenue, NW, Washington, DC 20001.

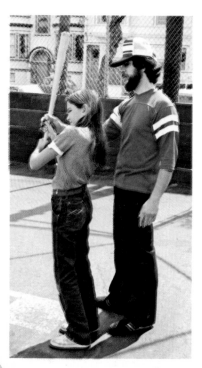
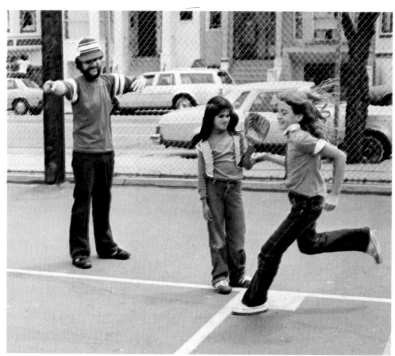

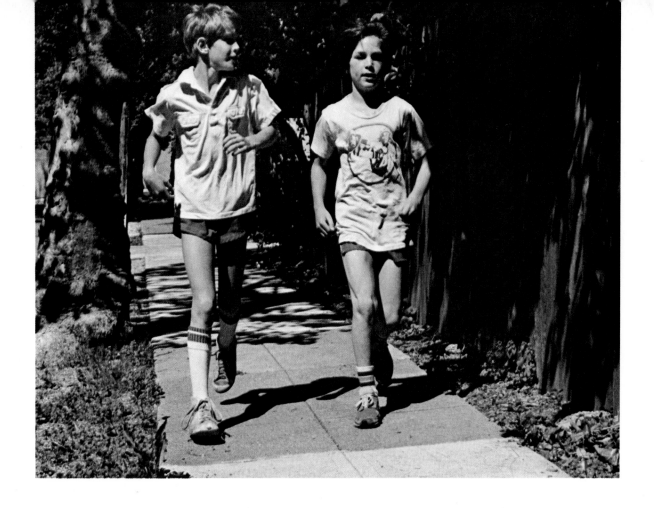

EXERCISING SAFELY

Maybe you want to exercise more to help your muscles, heart, and lungs. But it is not safe to begin doing a lot of exercise immediately. You must be careful to exercise safely.

How to Exercise

Some people need more exercise than others. Check with your doctor or school nurse to find out how much exercise is right for you. Then start out slowly and do just a little more exercise each day. After two or three months you will be able to exercise safely for a longer time.

How might these boys have begun their exercise program safely?

Talking About Exercise

With a friend, talk about how you can exercise safely at school and at home.

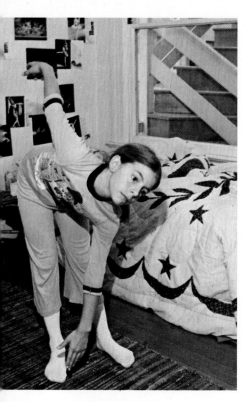

Is this girl exercising safely? How can you tell?

Where and When to Exercise

Before you exercise, find a place where you will have room to move around. Do not exercise right after eating or right before bedtime. Exercise at these times makes it hard for you to digest your food or to fall asleep. You should exercise at the time of day when you feel most active and alert.

Kinds of Exercise

Active games are good exercise for your body. Basketball and soccer make your arm and leg muscles work hard. They also make you breathe hard and make your heart beat fast.

You should do some exercises to warm up and stretch before you play active games. The exercises help get your muscles, heart, and lungs ready to work hard.

The exercises in the back of this book can get you ready for active games. These exercises help your heart, your lungs, and the muscles in different parts of your body. Read the directions carefully. Then try to do the exercises. Start slowly and exercise safely. If you do some of these exercises each day, you can help all of your body's muscles become stronger.

REVIEW IT NOW

1. How should you begin if you want to start exercising more?
2. What should you do before playing any active game?

Fitness With Gymnastic Equipment

Many people stretch, swing, and jump during play. Some enjoy playing on gymnastic equipment such as the balance beam and the parallel bars. Playing on this equipment can help keep the body fit and improve balance and coordination.

Exercising on the balance beam can improve a person's balance. Some gymnasts even turn exercise on the balance beam into art by doing movements almost perfectly. The parallel bars can strengthen the muscles in the arms and back. Coordination can improve, too.

Using gymnastic equipment can help strengthen muscles. These muscles then can work together for fitness.

Health Today

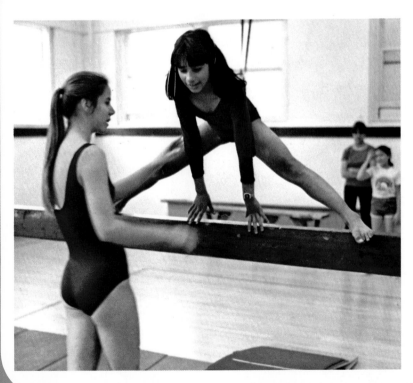

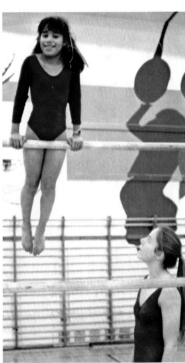

RESTING AND SLEEPING TO STORE ENERGY

Kiyo has had a very busy day. Her body has been working all the time. Now she is asleep. Her body is resting. But it has not stopped working. It is still using energy, but less than when she was awake. Kiyo's body is working to store energy for her next busy day.

Kiyo's body worked hard during her busy day. But even when Kiyo sleeps, her body is working. What work is her body doing?

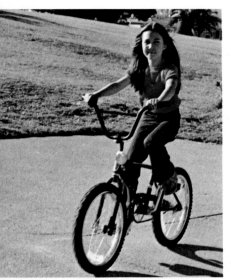
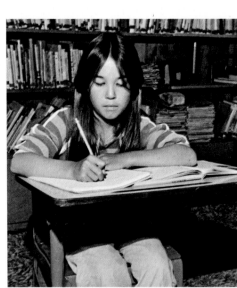
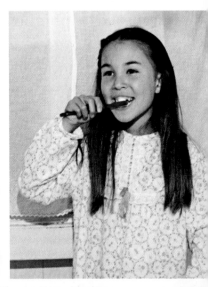

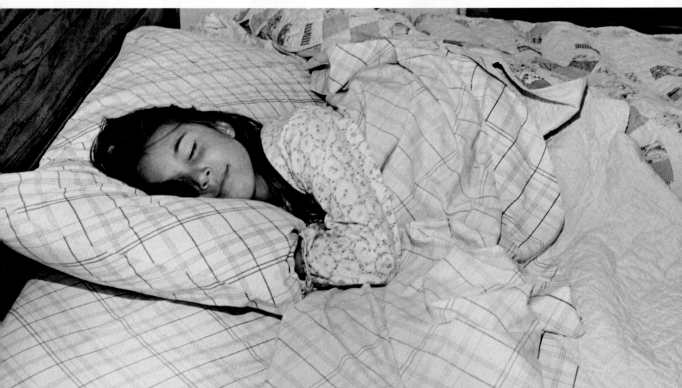

Resting

When your body has worked long or hard, you start to feel tired. Sometimes your muscles feel sore. You begin to slow down. You may start to feel sleepy.

Tired feelings help your body protect itself. They keep your body from working too hard. They let you know that your body needs to rest.

When you rest, your body systems slow down and use less energy. Sitting quietly is one way you can rest. Another way is by sleeping.

Sleeping

When you sleep, your body and your brain rest. Scientists do not know exactly why people need to sleep. But everyone must sleep for part of each day. If people go without sleep for a few days, they become ill.

What Happens During Sleep?

Many things happen in your body while you sleep. Your nerve cells are less active. Your heart slows down. When you sleep, you do not breathe as often as when you are awake. Your body repairs many of its parts while you sleep.

When you sleep, your body uses less energy than when you are awake and active. It stores the nutrients in food you will need for energy. When you wake up in the morning, you feel rested. You have the energy you need for the day's activities.

Resting to Relax

Many times your muscles tighten up. They can feel tired or sore. Resting helps your muscles relax. They loosen up and help your whole body relax.

Your Body's Clock

Many scientists believe that we have something that works like a clock inside our brain. This "clock" tells our bodies when to sleep and when to wake up.

Wellness Tip

Sleep either on your side or on your back. Sleeping on your stomach is not healthful for your back. It may cause too much strain on your spine and back muscles.

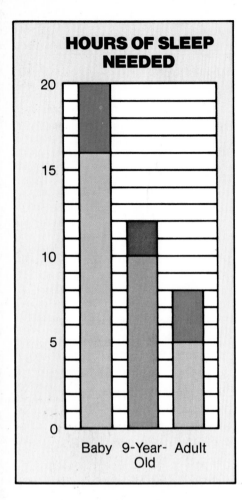

HOURS OF SLEEP NEEDED

20
15
10
5
0

Baby 9-Year- Adult
        Old

How many hours of sleep does a nine-year-old child need?

The amount of sleep a person needs depends partly on age. When you were a baby, you needed more sleep than you do now. Most people your age need about eleven hours of sleep. Some adults need only five or six hours of sleep each night.

One reason you need more sleep than older people is that you are more active. Another reason is that you are still growing. You need a lot of energy to be active and to grow. You need to sleep a lot so that you can store all the energy your body needs.

As you become older, your body stops growing larger. You may not be as active as you are now, either. You will need less sleep than you do now.

By getting regular exercise and enough sleep, you are helping yourself reach wellness.

REVIEW IT NOW

1. How do tired feelings help your body protect itself?
2. What happens to your body when you sleep?
3. About how much sleep do people your age need?
4. Why do you need more sleep than an older person does?

Planning a Fitness Field Day

You and your family or friends can organize your own "Fitness Field Day." Have each person make up a fitness exercise or event. There should be no winners or losers. The object is to get physical exercise and have fun.

As you plan, answer these questions:

- Are warm-up exercises needed first?
- How will the exercise or event help the body?
- What muscles will be used?

Be sure that each exercise and event in your field day is one that every person can do. Then everyone can exercise safely—and have fun!

Working Toward Wellness

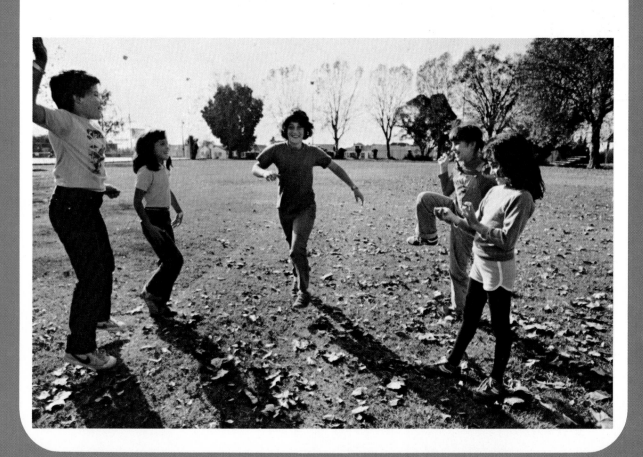

To Help You Review

Checking Your Understanding

Write the numbers from 1 to 12 on your paper. After each number, write the answer to the question or questions. Page numbers in ( ) tell you where to look in the chapter if you need help.

1. What are three ways that regular exercise helps your body? (**108**)
2. How does exercise help your body use the food you eat? (**109**)
3. What are three ways that exercises such as swimming or dancing help your muscles? (**110**)
4. What are four ways that good posture helps your body? (**112**)
5. Where do the muscles get the extra energy they need during exercise? (**115**)
6. What happens to your pulse if you do regular exercise? Why? (**117**)
7. What kinds of exercise help your heart and lungs the most? (**118**)
8. Why should you not exercise right after eating or right before bedtime? (**122**)
9. What are two reasons you should do warm-up exercises before you play active games? (**122**)
10. How do tired feelings help your body protect itself? (**125**)
11. What are four things that happen in your body while you sleep? (**125**)
12. Why do young people often need more sleep than adults? (**126**)

Checking Your Health Vocabulary

Write the numbers from 1 to 3 on your paper. After each number, write the letter of the meaning for the word. Page numbers in ( ) tell you where to look in the chapter if you need help.

1. exercise (**108**)   **2.** posture (**112**)   **3.** pulse (**117**)

a. the push of blood through your arteries with each heartbeat
b. any activity that makes your body work hard
c. the way you hold your body

Write the numbers from 4 to 10 on your paper. Read each sentence and fill in the missing word. The first letter of each missing word is given. Page numbers in ( ) tell you where to look in the chapter if you need help.

4. Regular exercise makes your heart and m_____ strong. (**108**)
5. Exercise helps your body use f_____. (**109**)
6. Good posture helps your l_____ get plenty of air. (**112**)
7. Your heart beats faster than normal during e_____. (**114**)
8. Your lungs take in more o_____ when you exercise. (**115**)
9. Feeling tired lets you know your body needs to r_____. (**125**)
10. When you s_____, your body and brain rest. (**125**)

Practice Test

True or False?

Write the numbers from 1 to 15 on your paper. After each number, write *T* if the sentence is *true*. Write *F* if it is *false*. Rewrite each false sentence to make it true.

1. Regular exercise is not important if you eat a balanced diet.
2. Exercise helps your body turn the nutrients from food into fat.
3. Some exercises make your muscles able to work a long time without becoming tired.
4. Good posture helps your body work at its best.
5. When you exercise, your cells quickly use food for energy.
6. Carbon dioxide is a waste your cells make.
7. Your body uses less oxygen when you exercise.
8. With regular exercise, your heart can pump more blood.
9. Exercises such as swimming and jumping rope help your heart and lungs the most.
10. You should exercise right before going to bed.
11. You should do exercises to warm up before you play active games.
12. If people go without sleep for a few days, they will be healthy.
13. Your heart slows down when you sleep.
14. Most young people need about seven hours of sleep.
15. Adults who do not exercise often need less sleep than a young person who exercises a lot.

Complete the Sentence

Write the numbers from 16 to 20 on your paper. After each number, copy the sentence and fill in the missing word.

16. If your _____ work hard every day, they will hold more air.
17. _____ muscles can cause poor posture.
18. Your _____ carries oxygen to your cells and carries away wastes.
19. You should start out _____ when you begin to exercise.
20. When you sleep, your body uses less _____.

Learning More

For You to Do

1. Write to the President's Council on Physical Fitness and Sports, 400 6th Street SW, Washington, DC 20201. Ask about exercises a person your age could do to have a healthy body.

2. List places in your neighborhood or near your school where you could play active games safely. Then make a map that shows where these places are. You also might draw a line to show how to get to each place safely from your home.

3. Write down how many hours of sleep you get each night. Do this for a week. Add up the figures, then divide by seven. How many hours of sleep do you get on the average each night. How do you know that you are getting enough sleep? Not enough sleep?

For You to Find Out

1. Choose a sport you like. Ask your physical education teacher what exercises a person should do to warm up before playing this sport.

2. What are the Olympic games? When did they start? Who plays in them? What are some games and contests in the Olympics? Use an encyclopedia to find out.

3. What are dreams? During which part of sleep do people usually dream? Use library books about sleep or dreams to help you find out.

For You to Read

Here are some books you can look for in your school or public library to find out more about exercise and sleep.

Cosgrove, Margaret. *Your Muscles and Ways to Exercise Them.* Dodd, 1980.

Goodbody, Slim. *The Force Inside You.* Coward-McCann, 1983.

Trier, Carola. *Exercise: What It Is, What It Does.* Greenwillow, 1982.

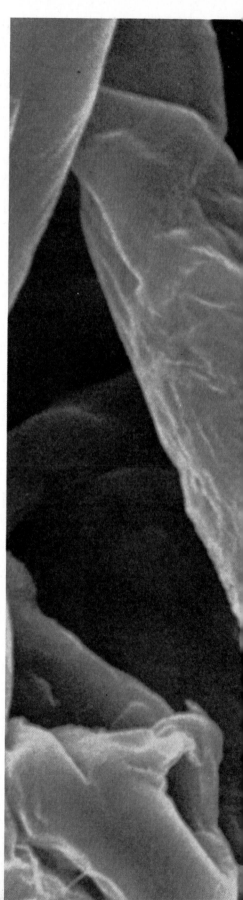

CHAPTER 6

Guarding Against Disease Microbes

Have you ever heard someone say, "I had a bug"? That is how some people say they were ill. They did not really have bugs in their bodies. But they did have another kind of tiny creature.

These creatures, which are too small to see with only your eyes, can enter your body and make you ill. Your body works to keep these creatures out. If you get "a bug," your body works to get rid of it.

There are ways you can help keep from becoming ill. Practicing good health habits is one way. Even when you have wellness, your body needs your help to fight illness.

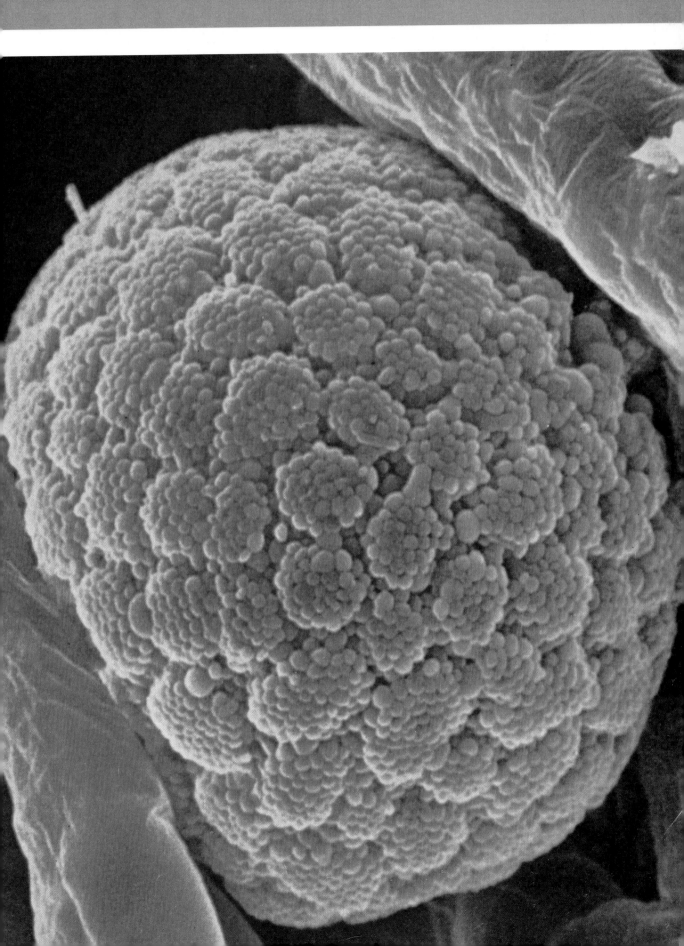

Thinking About Symptoms

Think about the last time you were ill. What disease did you have? What were its symptoms? Try to remember at least three symptoms.

WHY DO PEOPLE GET SICK?

Sally Ritt is ill today. She has a cough and a sore throat. She has no energy and her body feels hot. She has the flu.

Sally has a **disease.** A disease is any breakdown in the way the body works. It means that some part of the body has stopped working as it should.

Disease can make a person feel discomfort and pain. It may cause other signs as well. The pains and other signs of a disease are called its **symptoms.** Each disease has its own set of symptoms. The symptoms of a cold, for example, may include a runny nose, a cough, and a sore throat.

When you have the symptoms of a disease, you should see a doctor. Some diseases have the same symptoms. Only a doctor can tell you if you need medicine or if your body is strong enough to get rid of the disease by itself.

Why is Sally staying in bed today?

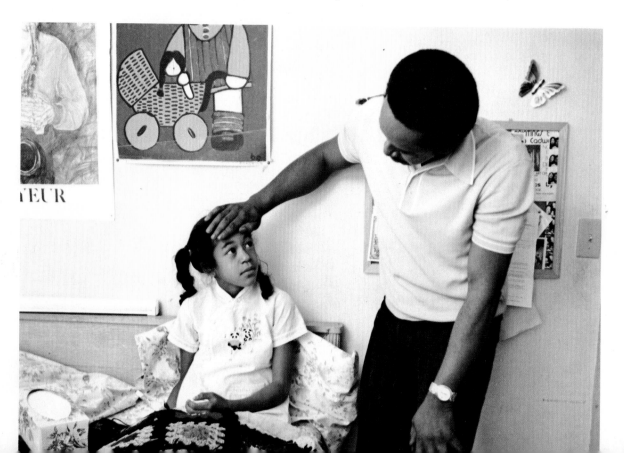

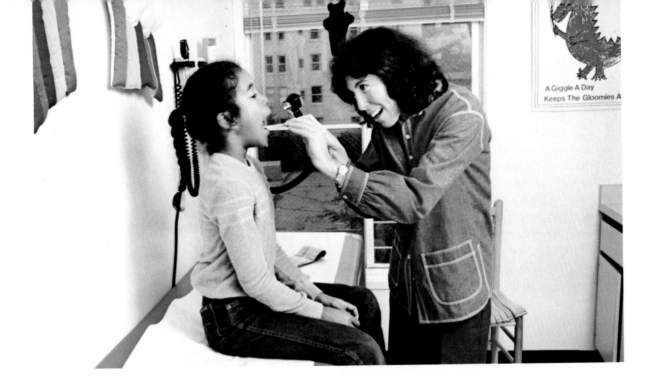

Some diseases can pass from one person to another. These are called **communicable diseases.** They are caused by tiny living creatures called microbes.

Microbes are so small that they cannot be seen without a microscope. Thousands of microbes would fit in a single drop of water. Some microbes are helpful to human beings. Some are harmless. Many other kinds, however, cause disease.

Why should you see a doctor when you have the symptoms of a disease?

Other Kinds of Disease

Some kinds of disease are not passed from one person to another. They are **noncommunicable diseases.** Scientists do not know the causes of many of these diseases. But some can be caused by unhealthful living habits. People may get a noncommunicable disease if they do not have a balanced diet or if they do not get enough exercise or sleep. Noncommunicable diseases include heart disease and cancer.

Different Kinds of Microbes

Microbes live almost everywhere. Some live in water. Others live in soil or air. Some even live on or in your body without harming you. Some of these microbes are needed for the body systems to work properly.

All microbes belong to four main groups. Each group includes some harmless microbes, as well as some that can cause disease.

Bacteria

One group of microbes is called **bacteria.** Bacteria are very small. A line of 1,000 bacteria could fit inside the period at the end of this sentence. The pictures show the different shapes of bacteria.

Bacteria can live almost anywhere. All bacteria need food and water to stay alive. Some bacteria also need air. But others can live without it. Some bacteria need warmth. Others can live only where it is cold. Bacteria live wherever they can get the things they need to stay alive.

Bacteria have three basic shapes. What shapes are shown here?

© Carolina Biological Supply Company

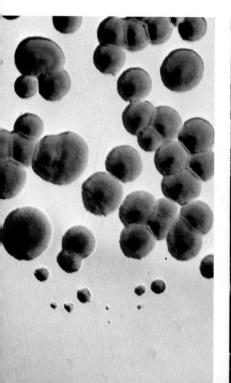
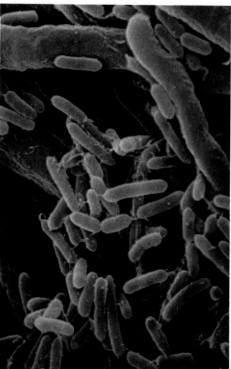
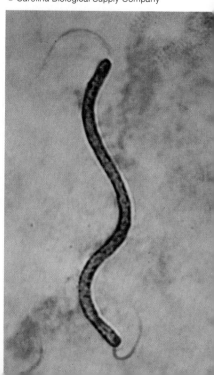

Viruses

The microbes in another group are called **viruses.** These are the smallest kind of microbe.

Most of the time viruses do not grow, change, or move. Some scientists are not sure if viruses are alive. But viruses can move into cells. Then they act as if they were alive.

Viruses can live in all kinds of cells. They can live in plant cells, animal cells, or human cells. They can even live inside bacteria. But any one type of virus can live in only certain kinds of cells.

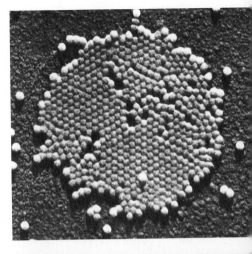

Fungi

Another group of microbes is called **fungi.** They cannot move by themselves. But if they land in the right place, they can grow and increase in number.

Many fungi are small. Often they live together in large groups. Fungi do not need light in order to live. Some fungi grow best in warm, wet places. Others grow best in dry, dusty places. Some fungi grow on or inside the human body.

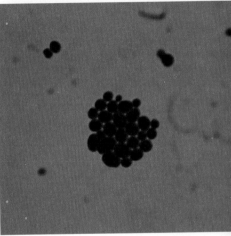

Protozoa

The fourth group of microbes is called **protozoa.** They need food and water to stay alive. Protozoa can move about on their own. They can find and eat their own food.

Protozoa are the largest kind of microbe. They usually live in ponds, streams, and other wet places. A few can live inside people.

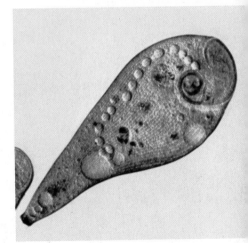

© Carolina Biological Supply Company

What differences can you see in the viruses, fungi, and protozoa?

You have microbes living inside your body all the time. Most of these microbes are harmless. They help to keep your body working well, too.

How Microbes Cause Disease

Sometimes microbes can cause disease when they enter your body. These are called **disease microbes.** They can enter through your nose or your mouth. They can enter through cuts and scratches in your skin.

A small number of disease microbes inside your body cannot harm you. But if the microbes increase in number, they can make you ill.

How can disease microbes enter your body?

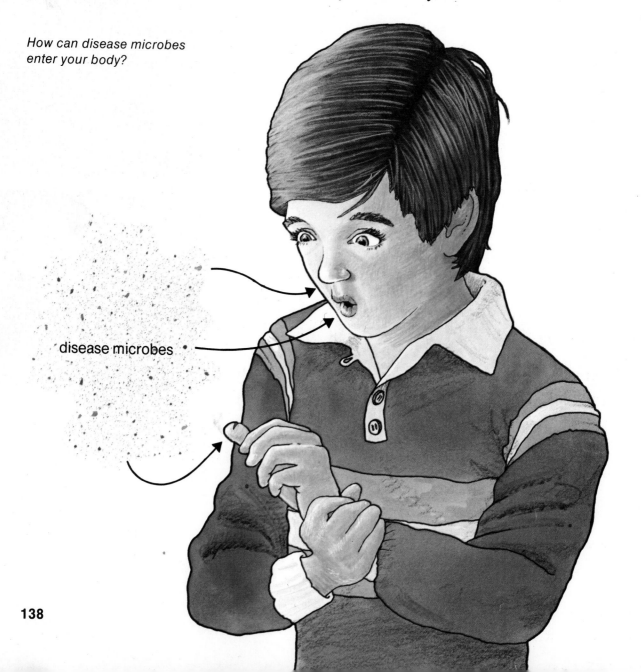

disease microbes

138

How Microbes Grow

Bacteria, fungi, and protozoa are all cells. They use food to grow larger. When they reach a certain size, they divide in two. Each part becomes a new cell. Both new cells use food to grow. Then they also divide. They become four new cells.

Look at the pictures to see how one cell divides into two. It divides again and again. This is just what disease microbes do inside your body.

Viruses are not cells. They cannot divide the same way cells do. But viruses, too, have a way to increase in number. When a virus gets inside a living cell, it takes control of the cell. It makes the cell stop doing its usual work. The cell starts making new viruses instead. At last the cell is full of viruses. Then it splits open. The viruses spill out and enter other nearby cells. Each of these cells makes more viruses. In this way, one virus soon turns into many viruses.

How Microbes Can Harm You

When you have many disease microbes in your body, you have an **infection.** An infection is the growth of disease microbes somewhere inside your body. Microbes can harm you in different ways. Some microbes make poisons. The poisons make you ill. Other microbes use up nutrients meant for your cells. Then your tissues are harmed. Some of your organs may stop working as they should. The infection in your body becomes a disease.

Different kinds of microbes cause different diseases. One kind of virus, for example, causes measles. Viruses cause the many different kinds of flu. Each kind is caused by a different type of virus.

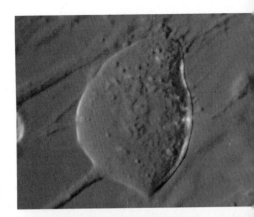
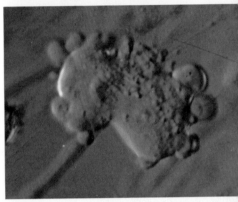
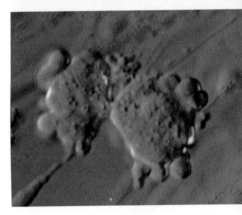

What will happen to this disease microbe after it divides into two?

139

A certain kind of bacteria causes strep throat. Look at the chart of some communicable diseases caused by microbes. Notice that each disease is caused by a different kind of microbe.

MICROBES	DISEASES
Viruses	common cold flu polio measles
Bacteria	strep throat tuberculosis
Protozoa	malaria dysentery
Fungi	athlete's foot ringworm

REVIEW IT NOW

1. What is a disease?
2. What is a communicable disease?
3. What are the four main groups of microbes?
4. What are disease microbes?
5. What is an infection?

Health Scientist

Diseases often are mysteries. Many times we do not know where they come from or how they spread. A *health scientist* works to find out how people get a disease, how it is spread, and how it can be controlled.

Many health scientists work in laboratories studying disease microbes. Others travel to areas where a disease has broken out. They search for clues to the cause of the disease.

Health scientists need at least four years of college training. To learn more about being a health scientist, write to the Centers for Disease Control, 1600 Clifton Road NE, Atlanta, GA 30333.

Health
Career

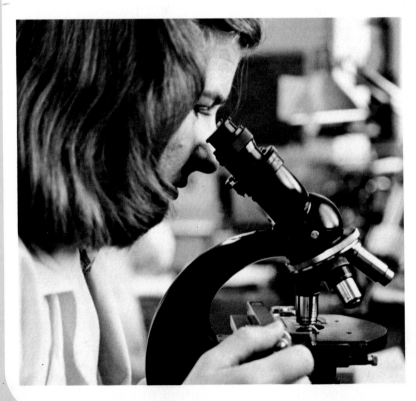
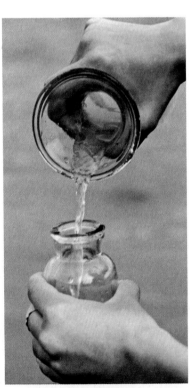

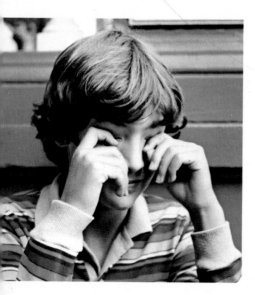

How can Neil help prevent his eye infection from spreading to others?

AVOIDING DISEASE MICROBES

Disease can spread in many different ways. But disease microbes can harm you only if they get inside your body. Once you find out how microbes spread, you can keep most of the harmful ones out of your body.

People Can Spread Disease

People with communicable diseases have many microbes in their bodies and on their skin. They can leave microbes behind on anything they touch. The microbes can get on your skin if you touch the same things. Then the microbes can get inside your body and make you ill.

Neil had an eye infection. The infection was caused by bacteria. His eyes felt itchy, so he rubbed them. The harmful bacteria got onto his hands. Then they got onto the chalk, the doorknobs, and the other things he touched.

Many of Neil's classmates touched these same objects. They got bacteria on their fingers. Then they touched their eyes and faces. Within a few days, many of Neil's classmates had itchy eyes.

People who are ill can also breathe, sneeze, or cough harmful microbes into the air. If you are nearby, you may breathe that air. Then the microbes can get into your lungs and make you ill.

You should try to stay away from people with communicable diseases. Do not share their food, silverware, plates, glasses, or cups. Try not to touch things they have touched. This will help to keep their disease microbes from spreading to you.

Medicines and Disease

The flu is a disease that people can spread. The flu caused more deaths in 1900 than any other disease. Now it causes far fewer deaths. That is because scientists found out how the flu virus harms people and how it spreads. They made medicines that help prevent people from getting the flu.

142

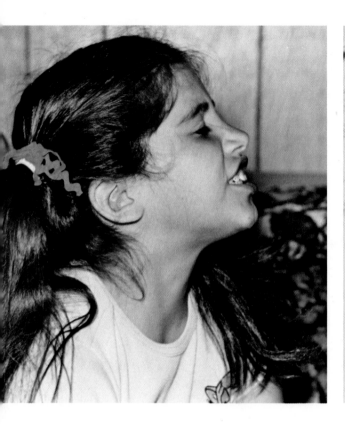
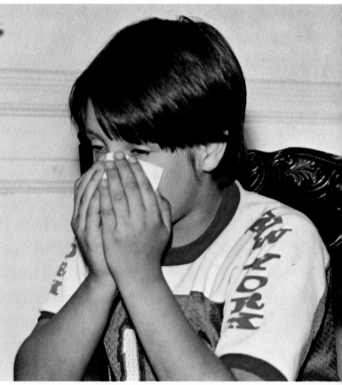

Suppose you become ill. You can avoid passing your disease to others. You can stay home until you are well. You can be careful not to share your food with anyone. You can make sure to wash your hands often. And you can cover your mouth with a tissue when you cough or sneeze.

The girl shown here is spreading disease microbes as she sneezes. The boy is not. Why?

Water Can Spread Disease

Many disease microbes grow very well in warm, dirty water. Some can stay alive for a long time even in cold water. Water in a pond or lake probably contains many microbes.

If you drink this water, it can make you ill. If the water is very dirty, even swimming in it can be risky. Microbes can get into cuts in your skin. Or you may swallow some of the water by mistake.

Finding Out About Your Drinking Water

Where does your drinking water at home come from? What was done to make it safe to drink?

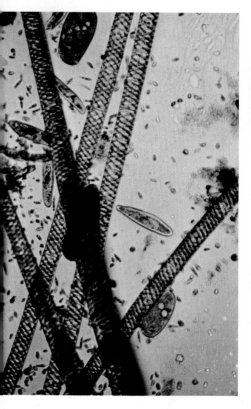

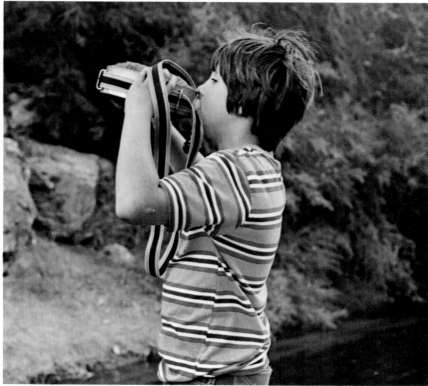

In what way has Howie prevented these disease microbes from entering his body?

Ray and Howie went for a hike. It was a hot day, and the boys became thirsty. They came to a stream. The water looked clear and clean. Ray wanted to take a drink. But Howie talked him out of it.

Howie told Ray to take a drink from his canteen. Howie had filled the canteen at home before he left. The water was a little warm, but it was free of harmful microbes.

You can avoid many diseases by drinking only water that you know is safe. Your water at home comes from a safe water supply. The microbes in it have been killed. All the dirt and harmful substances have been taken out. This makes the water safe to drink.

Food Can Spread Disease

Sometimes harmful microbes grow on food. They can make the food smell or look bad. Eating that food can make you ill.

Microbes can also cause food to spoil. Food spoils when it is left out in the warm air for a few hours. Foods such as meat, chicken, milk, and eggs spoil very easily. Eating spoiled food can make you ill.

One sunny day last July, Springville had a picnic. People ate lots of hamburgers and potato salad. The potato salad was made with mayonnaise. Mayonnaise has eggs in it.

The potato salad was left in the hot sun. About four hours later, Anita noticed that it was still there. She knew the mayonnaise in the salad might have spoiled by then. It was no longer safe to eat. She threw it out so that no one would eat any of it by mistake.

Storing food properly helps keep it safe. Store any food that may spoil in the refrigerator. If some foods are left out for a long time, they should not be eaten.

Some foods may have harmful microbes or chemicals on them when you buy them. The chemicals may have been sprayed on them to keep insects away. You should always wash fruits and vegetables before you eat them.

You should eat only food that you know is safe. If any food smells or looks bad to you, do not eat it. Never eat any food that has mold on it.

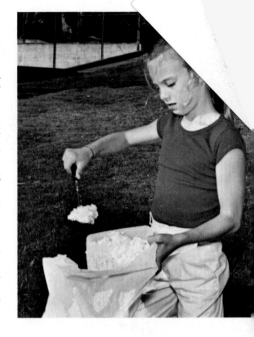

How might Anita have prevented disease from spreading?

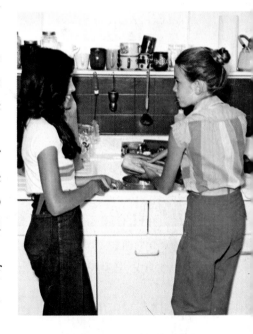

Why are these two girls washing the vegetables before making dinner?

145

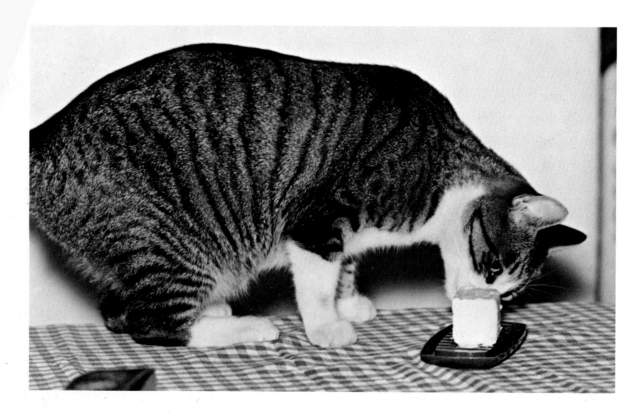

Is this butter safe to eat? Why or why not?

Animals and Insects Can Spread Disease

Some microbes are carried by animals. A sick animal is more likely to spread disease than a healthy animal. But even healthy animals carry microbes in their mouths. Often these microbes are harmless to the animal. But they can make people very ill.

Sue was setting the table. Her cat jumped up and licked the butter. Sue threw the butter away. Her cat is clean, but she knows that any cat has microbes in its mouth. The microbes may have gotten on the butter when the cat licked it. Some of these microbes may have been disease microbes.

You should stay away from strange animals. Do not pet dogs or cats that you do not know. Never try to pick up a squirrel that lets you come close. If an animal ever bites you, tell an adult at once. You may have to see a doctor quickly.

Finding Out About Rabies

Rabies is a disease that can be spread by animal bites. How can you and your friends avoid this disease?

Insects spread many harmful diseases, too. Mosquitoes, fleas, and ticks can carry disease microbes in their bodies. If they sting or bite you, they put microbes into your body. Many harmful insects live in swamps and in dirty places. You should stay away from such places.

Houseflies do not bite or sting. But they are often covered with harmful microbes. They shake off some of these microbes wherever they go. Never let flies land on your food or on anything else you may put in your mouth.

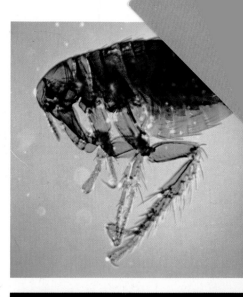

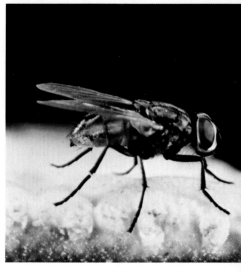

What are two ways insects can spread disease?

HOW MICROBES SPREAD	HOW TO STOP THEM
Animal bites	Do not touch strange animals.
Coughing and sneezing	Throw away tissues. Cover mouth and nose.
Water	Boil water when camping. Use tap water.
Food	Do not eat food that smells bad. Store food properly.

REVIEW IT NOW

1. What are four ways people spread disease microbes?
2. How can you avoid disease microbes in water?
3. When can food spoil?
4. What is one way to avoid diseases spread by animals?

A New Disease Control

Health Today

Mosquitoes sometimes spread dangerous diseases. But now scientists are working with a bacteria they call *BTI.* It kills mosquitoes.

Just like all living things, bacteria need food to live. Scientists think that when BTI cannot get enough food, it makes a deadly substance. When mosquitoes eat this BTI, the deadly substance enters their bodies. It kills the mosquitoes.

In experiments, the BTI is spread over small areas of land where mosquitoes live. All living things are watched carefully. So far, only mosquitoes have died. The experiments have made scientists hopeful that they have found a safe way to control some diseases.

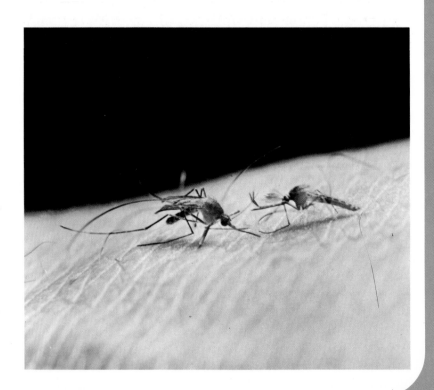

YOUR BODY CAN FIGHT DISEASE

Some microbes reach your body no matter what you do. In fact, hundreds of them reach you every day. Few of these microbes get inside you, however. And not all the ones that get inside you make you ill. Even when you do become ill, your body usually gets rid of the disease by itself. That is because your body has many ways to fight against microbes. These are called your body's **defenses.**

Your Outer Defenses

Most of the microbes that reach you stay on your skin. Your skin is your body's main outer defense. It keeps microbes from getting inside you. Washing your skin gets rid of these microbes.

Microbes can enter your skin through cuts and scratches. That is why you should wash any cut and cover it with a bandage. This keeps out harmful microbes while your cut is healing.

When you cut yourself, your skin makes its own bandage. The blood on the cut dries and forms a hard covering called a **scab.** When the skin beneath the scab has healed, the scab will fall off. New skin has closed up the cut.

Your Inner Defenses

If microbes get inside your body, your body's inner defenses go to work. White blood cells attack the harmful microbes. If they cannot destroy the microbes, your body has another defense.

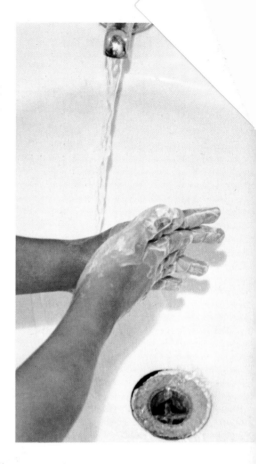

How does washing your skin help fight against disease?

Wellness Tip
Even though a scab may itch, it is important not to scratch it. The scab protects the area that is healing. Microbes cannot enter the cut. The new skin that is growing under the scab is protected from any harm, too.

How do white blood cells destroy harmful microbes?

White Blood Cells

White blood cells attack and destroy disease microbes in your body. They destroy harmful microbes by digesting them.

You have white blood cells in your blood all the time. They catch and destroy disease microbes inside you. If you get an infection, your body makes more white blood cells. Your blood carries the white blood cells to the infection. The white blood cells start to destroy the microbes.

Antibodies

Sometimes there are so many microbes that your white blood cells cannot destroy them fast enough. The microbes continue to increase in number. The infection spreads and makes you ill. Then your body uses another defense against microbes. Your white blood cells make a substance called an **antibody.** Antibodies surround the microbes and stop them from acting. The microbes cannot get food or grow. They cannot harm you either. At last, the white blood cells digest them.

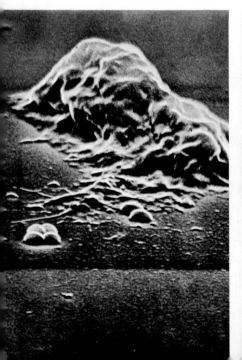
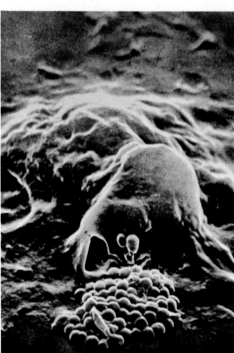
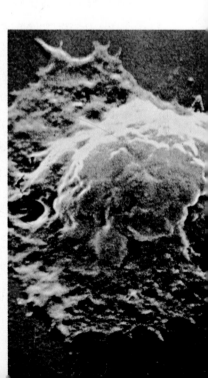

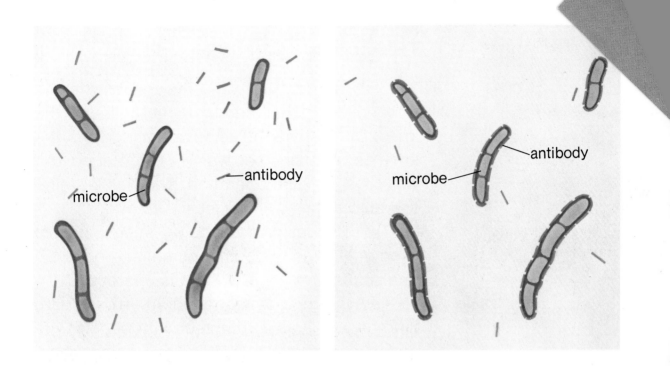

Each antibody acts against only one kind of microbe. It cannot act against any other kind. For example, if you have mumps, your body makes an antibody just for mumps. If you get chicken pox, your body makes a different antibody to fight the chicken pox microbes.

How do antibodies stop disease microbes from acting?

Some antibodies stay in your blood after you are well. Months or years later, microbes of the same kind may enter your body again. But this time your body is ready. Your body already has the antibodies it needs. They attack the harmful microbes right away. You have an **immunity** to the disease caused by those microbes. An immunity is your body's ability to defend itself with antibodies against microbes of a certain kind. The microbes cannot harm you again. When you have an immunity to a certain disease, you are **immune** to that disease.

Immunity to some diseases lasts a whole lifetime. Immunity to other diseases wears off after a while.

Focus On

Ted Kennedy, Jr.

Ted Kennedy, Jr., was 12 years old when he learned that he had cancer in his leg below the knee. Doctors had to remove his leg from the knee down. At first Ted was very frightened. But two days after the operation, Ted was learning to walk with an artificial leg.

Ted did not give up doing things that he liked or wanted to do. In fact, he learned to ski and scuba dive shortly after his operation.

Ted is now a college student. In his spare time he works as a volunteer with people who have diseases like his. Ted helps them understand the special problems they must face.

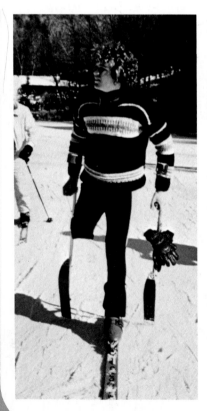
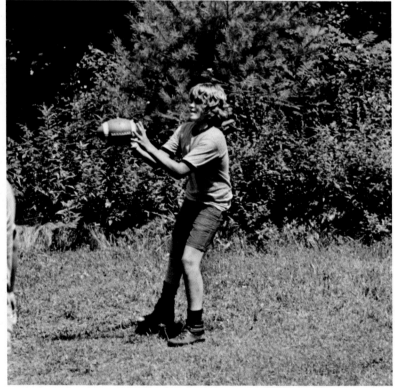

Building Up Your Defenses

You can help your body fight disease. Medicines called **vaccines** can help you form immunity to some diseases. Also, through healthful habits, you can build up your **resistance.** Resistance is your body's ability to fight off disease microbes.

Protecting Yourself With Vaccines

Becoming ill is one way to build immunity to a disease. But many diseases are very painful. Some are dangerous as well.

Vaccines help you build immunity to a disease without becoming ill. A vaccine puts a few microbes of a certain type into your blood. These microbes are too weak to make you ill. They may even be dead. But your body makes antibodies against them anyhow. The antibodies make you immune to that type of microbe. Then you cannot get the disease it normally causes.

Different vaccines protect you from different diseases. You need one kind of vaccine for polio and another kind for measles. Each kind of vaccine causes your body to make one kind of antibody. There are no vaccines for some diseases yet. For example, there is no vaccine for the common cold.

You can be **vaccinated,** or given a vaccine, in different ways. One vaccine may be something you swallow. Another may be given as a shot.

Some vaccines make you immune to a disease all your life. Others make you immune for a shorter time. You will need a **booster** of these vaccines. This means the doctor must give you the vaccine again. For some diseases, you may need a booster every few years.

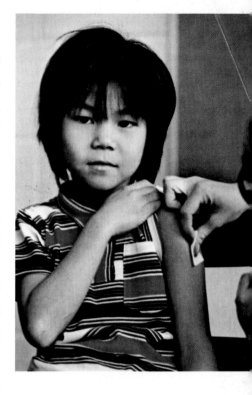

How do vaccines help you form an immunity?

Vaccines for Children

Many states have laws that say children must be vaccinated against certain diseases. The vaccines for these diseases usually are given in the early years of school. The school doctor may vaccinate you if you do not have a family doctor or if you cannot see your own.

Controlling Measles

Early in 1981, the Centers for Disease Control made a report about measles. The report said that the number of cases of measles has gone down. It also said that measles probably will be very rare in the United States by the end of 1982. Vaccinating children for measles has helped lower the number of cases of this disease.

Building Up Your Resistance

Vaccines make you immune only to certain diseases. But your body can fight against all diseases if it has resistance. Strong resistance means that your body easily can fight disease microbes.

Healthful habits can help you build up your resistance. You need a balanced diet. You need regular exercise and the right amount of sleep. You also can help your body fight disease by staying warm. If you have healthful habits, you are helping your body stay healthy and strong.

There are microbes everywhere you go. Most people have some disease microbes in their bodies all the time. You probably have some inside you right now. But as long as you stay strong and healthy, the microbes cannot make you ill.

REVIEW IT NOW

1. What is your body's main outer defense against disease microbes?
2. What are your body's two inner defenses against disease microbes?
3. What is immunity?
4. What are vaccines?
5. What is resistance?

Being a "Disease Detective"

To understand how easily disease microbes spread, you and your family can be "disease detectives" for a day.

Pretend that you have a communicable disease. Pay close attention to everything you do during the day. Watch for ways you can spread disease microbes to others. Have your family watch, too. Do you share food or drink? Do you sneeze or cough without covering your mouth?

At the end of the day, sit down with your family and make a list of all the ways you could have spread disease microbes to others. Then decide how you can prevent disease microbes from spreading.

Working Toward Wellness

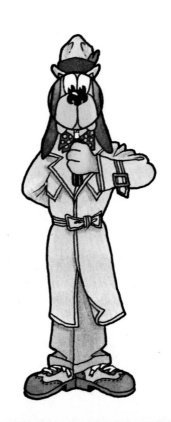

WAYS I CAN PREVENT DISEASE MICROBES FROM SPREADING

1. Do not share my food or drink.
2. Cover my mouth when I sneeze.
3. Wash my hands before I help make lunch or dinner.
4. Always throw away my tissues.

To Help You Review

Checking Your Understanding

Write the numbers from 1 to 14 on your paper. After each number, write the answer to the question. Page numbers in ( ) tell you where to look in the chapter if you need help.

1. What causes a communicable disease? (**135**)
2. What are three kinds of cells in which viruses can live? (**137**)
3. What three kinds of microbes are cells? (**139**)
4. What are four ways you can avoid spreading disease microbes to others? (**143**)
5. Why should you never drink water from a pond, stream, or lake? (**143**)
6. Why should foods such as meat, milk, and eggs be stored in the refrigerator? (**145**)
7. How do insects such as mosquitoes and fleas spread disease? (**147**)
8. What is your body's main outer defense? (**149**)
9. How does your skin form its own bandage? (**149**)
10. What inner defense goes to work as soon as disease microbes enter your body? (**149**)
11. How do antibodies act against disease microbes? (**150**)
12. What are two ways you can form immunity to some diseases? (**151, 153**)
13. When might you need a booster of a vaccine? (**153**)
14. What healthful habits can help your body build up strong resistance? (**154**)

Checking Your Health Vocabulary

Write the numbers from 1 to 6 on your paper. After each number, write the letter of the meaning for the word. Page numbers in ( ) tell you where to look in the chapter if you need help.

1. disease (**134**)   4. antibody (**150**)
2. symptoms (**134**)   5. vaccines (**153**)
3. defenses (**149**)   6. resistance (**153**)

a. ways your body has to fight against microbes
b. any breakdown in the way the body works
c. the body's ability to fight off disease microbes
d. medicines that help your body form immunity to some diseases
e. a substance the white blood cells make to stop a certain microbe from acting
f. pains and other signs of disease

Write the numbers from 7 to 12 on your paper. Then write a sentence that explains the meaning of each word or words. Page numbers in ( ) tell you where to look in the chapter if you need help.

7. communicable diseases (**135**)
8. disease microbes (**138**)
9. infection (**139**)
10. immunity (**151**)
11. immune (**151**)
12. vaccinated (**153**)

Practice Test

True or False?

Write the numbers from 1 to 15 on your paper. After each number, write *T* if the sentence is *true*. Write *F* if it is *false*. Rewrite each false sentence to make it true.

1. Communicable diseases can pass from one person to another.
2. Not all groups of microbes include disease microbes.
3. Fungi are the largest kind of microbe.
4. Bacteria, fungi, protozoa, and viruses grow by dividing again and again.
5. Different kinds of microbes cause different diseases.
6. Animals that are healthy cannot spread harmful microbes.
7. Microbes can enter your body only through your mouth or nose.
8. Washing your skin can get rid of many harmful microbes.
9. If you get an infection, your body makes more white blood cells.
10. Antibodies are made by your lungs.
11. Each antibody can act against many kinds of disease microbes.
12. If you are immune to a disease, the disease cannot harm you.
13. Immunity to all diseases lasts a lifetime.
14. There are no vaccines for some diseases.
15. Good health habits can build up your body's resistance.

Complete the Sentence

Write the numbers from 16 to 20 on your paper. After each number, copy the sentence and fill in the missing word.

16. The four main groups of microbes are bacteria, _____, fungi, and protozoa.
17. An infection is a growth of disease _____ somewhere in your body.
18. When you cut yourself, dried blood on the cut forms a _____.
19. _____ blood cells in your body attack and destroy disease microbes.
20. Some antibodies stay in your blood and help your body form an _____ to a disease.

Learning More

For You to Do

1. To see how microbes can grow in foods, try this activity. Find three containers that have tight lids. You can use bowls with plastic or foil wrap, too. In one, put a small piece of bread with a few drops of water. In the second, put a spoonful of cottage cheese. In the third, put a slice of an orange. Cover each container or bowl tightly. After 24 hours, check each one. Has the food changed in any way? Cover the containers again and leave them for two more days. How has the food changed?

2. Make a chart showing all the vaccines you have been given. For each vaccination, show:
   - what disease the vaccine protects against
   - how old you were when you got the vaccine (if you were vaccinated more than once, write down your age at each vaccination)
   - how you were vaccinated (by swallowing something, getting a shot, or another way)

For You to Find Out

1. What is "folk medicine?" What are some folk medicines that were used a hundred years ago? What are some folk medicines that people use today? You might ask a doctor or look in an encyclopedia to find out about folk medicine.

2. Dr. Jonas Salk invented a vaccine against a disease called polio in 1954. A few years later, in 1960, Dr. Albert Sabin invented another polio vaccine. Find out about polio and the first polio vaccines. Use an encyclopedia or library books about vaccines.

For You to Read

Here are some books you can look for in your school or public library to find out more about microbes and disease.

Berger, Melvin. *Germs Make Me Sick*. Crowell, 1985.

Knight, David C. *Viruses: Life's Smallest Enemies*. Morrow, 1981.

Nourse, Alan E. *Your Immune System*. Franklin Watts, 1982.

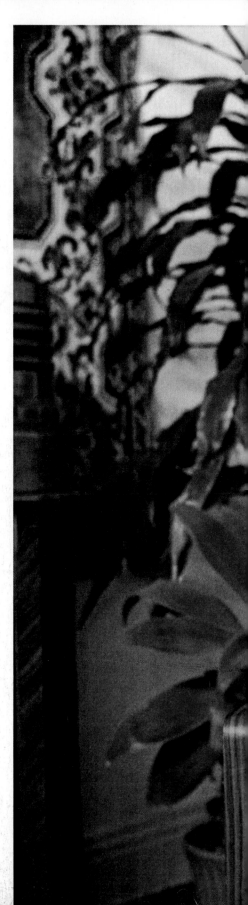

CHAPTER 7

Thinking About Drugs

Drugs can cause changes in your body. Many drugs help you feel better when you are ill. Some drugs, however, can put your wellness in danger.

You probably know that many people smoke tobacco and drink beverages that contain alcohol. But did you know that tobacco and drinks made with alcohol contain drugs that can put your wellness in danger?

Knowing about these and other drugs can help you make some important choices. Many of these choices can help you reach wellness.

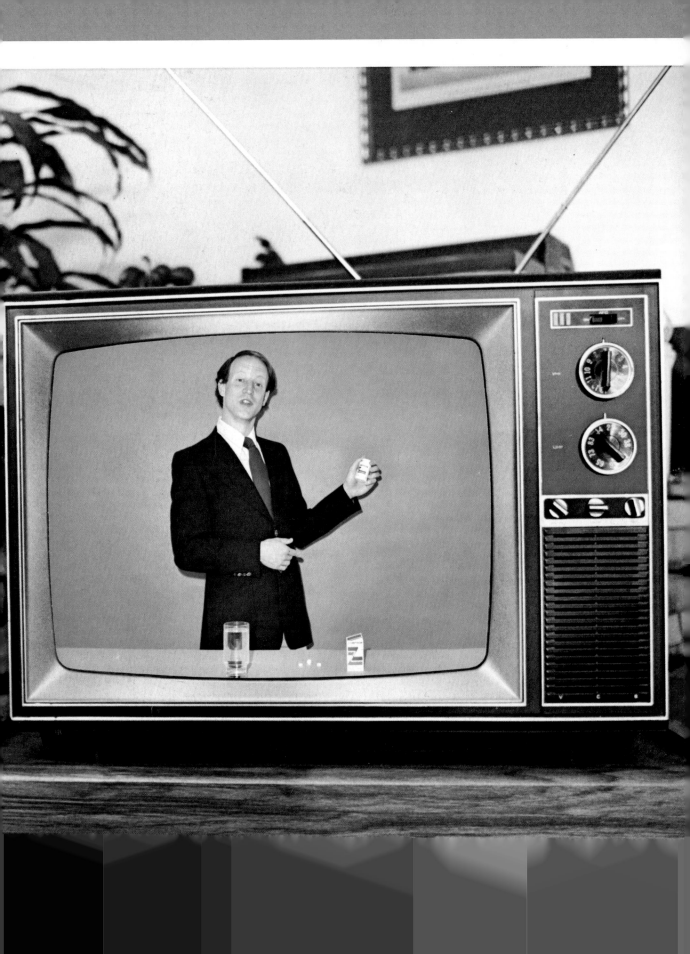

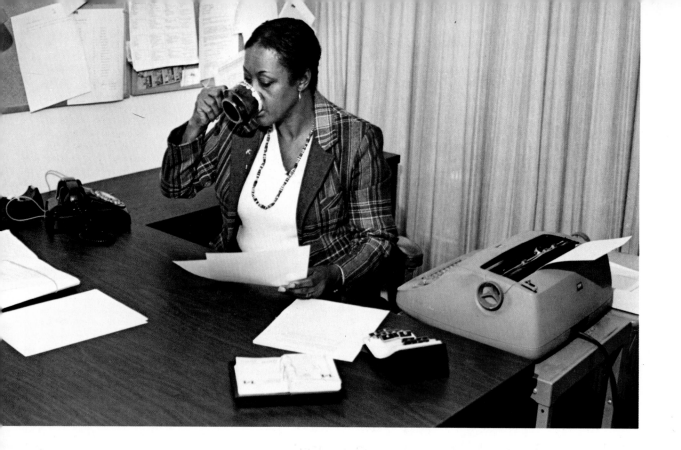

What substance does coffee contain that causes changes in Mrs. Hall's body?

Combining Drugs

Taking more than one drug at a time can be dangerous to your health. Each drug causes different changes in the body. If some of these changes happen at the same time, they can cause illness or even death. Always follow a doctor's orders when taking any drug.

HOW DRUGS CAN AFFECT YOU

Mrs. Hall drank something today that caused changes in her body. The drink made her heart beat faster. It made her blood vessels tighten up. It made Mrs. Hall feel more awake. Mrs. Hall drank a cup of coffee.

The coffee affected Mrs. Hall because coffee contains a **drug.** A drug is any substance other than food that causes changes in the body. There are many different kinds of drugs. For example, cold pills and cough syrup are drugs.

Each kind of drug causes different changes in the body. One drug may slow down the brain. Another may make the blood move faster. Most drugs cause more than one change at a time. Some drugs may cause different changes in different people.

Drugs That Can Help You

Some drugs can be used to help fight illness. These are called **medicines.** Suppose you have an illness and cannot get well by yourself. You may need a medicine to help your body fight the illness.

Lyle had a sore throat caused by bacteria in his body. The doctor gave him a medicine that helped kill the bacteria. Lyle followed the doctor's orders and took the medicine. He got well sooner than he thought he would.

Some medicines cannot help get rid of an illness. But they can make a person who is ill feel better for a while. They can get rid of the symptoms, or signs, of the illness.

Val had an illness called the flu. It made her whole body ache. The ache was one symptom of the flu. Val's mother gave her an aspirin–substitute medicine. The medicine was not meant to make Val's flu go away. It was to help ease Val's aches for a while. Val had to stay home and rest.

What might be some of the symptoms of the flu?

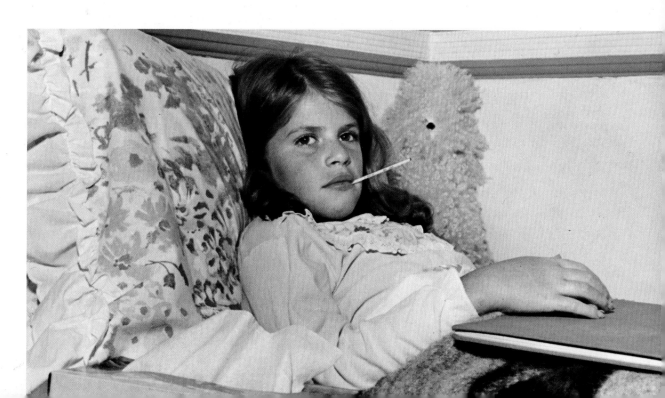

Taking Medicines Safely

All medicines should be taken with great care. You should always ask an adult before taking any medicine. The medicine may cause a number of changes in your body all at once. One of those changes may help you if you are ill. But other changes may be unneeded or unnecessary. These unneeded changes are called **side effects.**

Some cold medicines have side effects. They dry up a runny nose. But they may also make a person very sleepy. You should always find out the side effects of a medicine before you take it. Side effects are listed on the box or bottle that contains the medicine. You also can ask your doctor. Then you can use the medicine safely.

You should never take medicine unless you really need it. An adult should help you decide if you need the medicine. If you do need medicine, make sure to use it in the correct way. Medicines can do great harm when people use them incorrectly. For example, people sometimes take too much of a medicine. Or they take the medicine too often. Or they take the wrong medicine.

What warning about side effects is listed on this package?

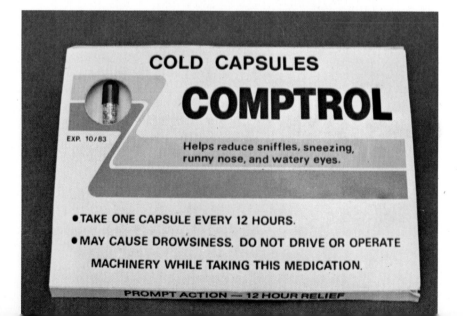

COLD CAPSULES

COMPTROL

EXP. 10/83

Helps reduce sniffles, sneezing, runny nose, and watery eyes.

● TAKE ONE CAPSULE EVERY 12 HOURS.

● MAY CAUSE DROWSINESS. DO NOT DRIVE OR OPERATE MACHINERY WHILE TAKING THIS MEDICATION.

PROMPT ACTION — 12 HOUR RELIEF

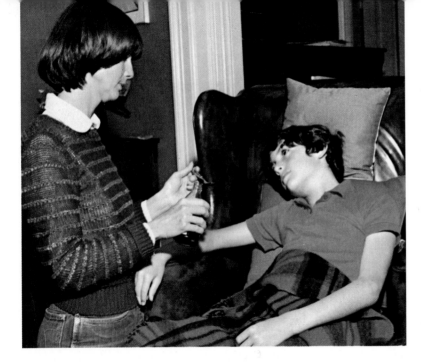

Why is it important to follow the directions exactly when taking a medicine?

You can avoid these mistakes by being careful. Every medicine comes with a set of directions. The directions tell you how to use the medicine. Follow the directions exactly when you take the medicine. If you feel any side effects, stop taking the medicine. Tell your doctor or an adult what happened.

Medicine Safety Rules

- Always check with an adult before taking any medicine.
- Do not use medicine unless you really need it.
- Do not use any prescription medicine unless your doctor tells you to.
- Read the directions each time you use a medicine.
- Always use medicine exactly the way the directions tell you to.
- Do not take two or more medicines at the same time unless your doctor tells you to.
- Throw out any medicine if you are not sure what it is.
- Keep all medicines out of the reach of children.

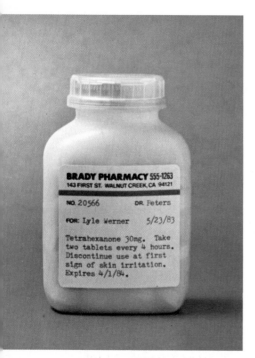

BRADY PHARMACY 555-1263
143 FIRST ST. WALNUT CREEK, CA 94121

NO. 20566   DR. Peters

FOR: Lyle Werner   5/23/83

Tetrahexanone 30mg. Take
two tablets every 4 hours.
Discontinue use at first
sign of skin irritation.
Expires 4/1/84.

Lyle needed a prescription medicine to help his sore throat.

Who prepares medicines that a doctor prescribes?

Prescription Medicines

Only a doctor can decide when some medicines should be used. These are called **prescription medicines.** They cannot be bought without an order, or **prescription,** from a doctor. A prescription is written for only one person. No other person should take the medicine.

When Lyle had a sore throat, his doctor gave him a prescription. Lyle and his father took the prescription to a drugstore near their home. They gave the prescription to the **pharmacist.** Pharmacists are specially trained workers who know how to prepare medicines.

The pharmacist prepared the medicine for Lyle. She made a prescription label for it that had Lyle's name on it. That meant only Lyle should take the medicine. The label also told how many pills Lyle should take and when to take them. It told him to stop using the medicine if he got a skin rash. It gave Lyle full directions for using the medicine.

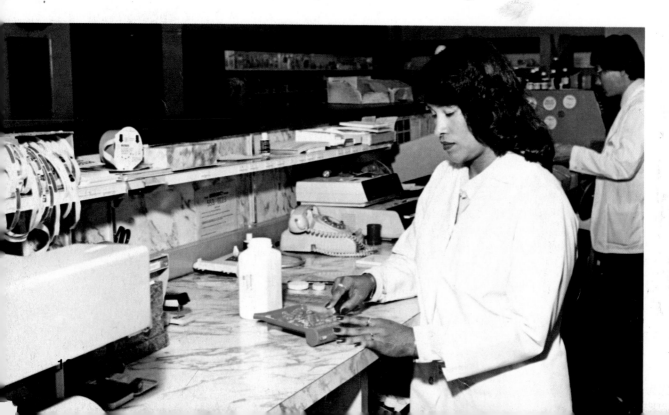

Over-the-Counter Medicines

Some medicines are called **over-the-counter medicines,** or **OTC medicines.** That means people can buy them without a prescription. The aspirin that Val's mother gave her is an OTC medicine. Val's father bought it in the food store.

OTC medicines usually are not as strong as prescription medicines. But they can still cause harm if they are used incorrectly. All OTC medicines have directions for using them. Before taking these medicines, be sure to read the directions. It tells what symptoms the medicine will help. It tells how much of the medicine to take and how often to take it. It warns you about the side effects the medicine may cause. It tells when to see a doctor instead of taking the medicine.

You should always ask an adult before taking any medicine. The directions tell the correct way to take the medicine. Follow the directions exactly when you use the medicine.

Wellness Tip

There may be OTC medicines in your home. How can you tell if they are still safe to use? Most OTC medicines can become unsafe after some time. With an adult, look at the date stamped on the labels of OTC medicines.

Why should you always read the label information on OTC medicines before buying them?

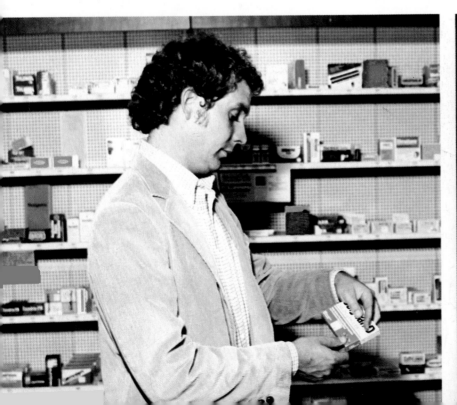

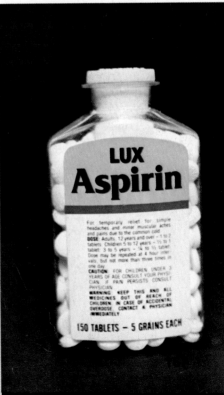

Physician

Health Career

It is hard to imagine the world without having even one *physician,* or doctor. Physicians perform a number of services that are important for health. They examine people and identify disease. They give medicines when a person is ill. Physicians also advise about diet and exercise to help keep the body healthy.

A person who wants to enter medical school to be a physician first must go to college for four years. Medical school usually takes four more years. To learn more about being a physician, write to the Council on Medical Education, American Medical Association, 535 North Dearborn Street, Chicago, IL 60610.

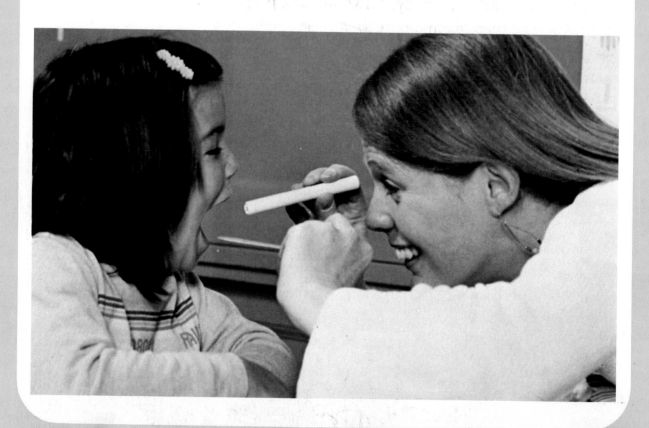

Drugs That Are Not Medicines

Many drugs cannot be used as medicines. They cannot help people who are ill. Sometimes these drugs have very strong effects. They can do great harm.

Caffeine

Mr. Ortega always has a cup of coffee with breakfast. It helps wake him up in the morning.

The part of coffee that helps Mr. Ortega wake up is **caffeine.** Caffeine is a drug found in cola drinks, chocolate, tea, and coffee. It speeds up the heart, the nerves, and many other parts of the body.

Most people can drink small amounts of coffee without damaging their health. But coffee can harm people who drink too much of it. A lot of coffee puts too much caffeine in the body. This can make people jittery. It can keep them awake when they want to fall asleep. Coffee has stronger effects on people with smaller bodies. That is why, at your age, it is best to drink no coffee at all.

Thinking About Coffee

Too much coffee can keep people awake. What else can too much coffee do to the body? How might too much coffee harm a person's health?

What is the drug in coffee that can make people jittery or keep them awake?

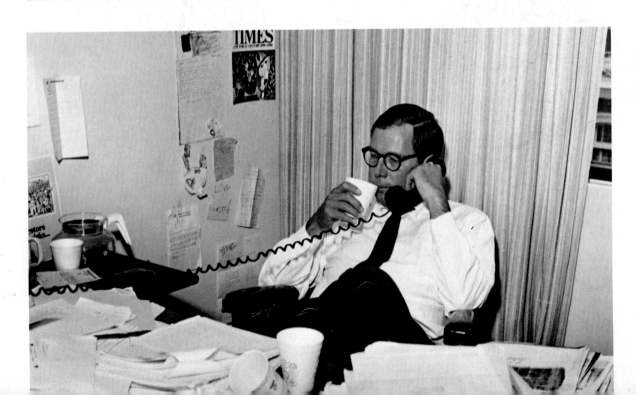

Finding Out About Alcohol and Tobacco

How many people in the United States drink alcohol? How many smoke cigarettes? A librarian may be able to help you find out.

Franz was watching a Western movie. One man in the movie drank some whiskey. When he tried to stand up, he fell over. He could not walk or talk properly. Everyone laughed at him. The man acted this way because of a drug in the whiskey. The drug is called **alcohol.** Alcohol is a drug found in drinks like beer, wine, and whiskey.

Some people use **tobacco,** but they do not smoke it. They use tobacco that can be put into the mouth and left there for a while. This type of tobacco is called **smokeless tobacco.** Chewing tobacco and dipping snuff are two kinds of smokeless tobacco. The drugs in smokeless tobacco are harmful to all parts of the mouth. Cancer of the mouth can result from using smokeless tobacco.

There are many harmful drugs like caffeine, alcohol, and those found in tobacco. These drugs cause great changes in a person's body. The changes cannot help solve any health problem and may even help cause some health problems.

REVIEW IT NOW

1. What is a drug?
2. What is a medicine?
3. What is a prescription drug?
4. What is an OTC medicine?
5. What is caffeine?
6. What is smokeless tobacco?

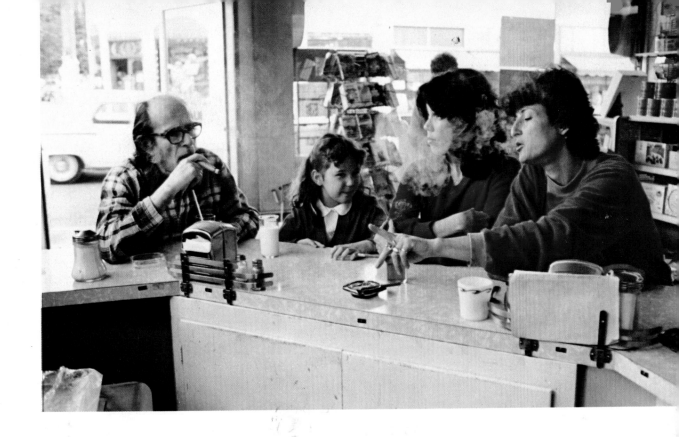

TOBACCO AND YOUR HEALTH

What are some ways people use tobacco?

Felice and her mother went to a coffee shop. Many people were smoking cigarettes. All of the tables had ashtrays. Some of the ashtrays were very full. Ashes were spilling out of them. The air smelled from tobacco smoke. Felice decided something right then. She decided never to smoke tobacco.

People use tobacco in many ways. Most people who use it smoke it in cigarettes. Other people smoke it in pipes or cigars.

Cigarettes may be the most harmful form of tobacco. That is because most people who smoke cigarettes breathe the smoke into their lungs. Drugs from the smoke then pass into their blood. Their blood carries the drugs to all their cells. The drugs cause changes in their whole body. The changes begin in less than a minute.

Harmful Smoke

Tobacco smoke can harm the health of a person who does not smoke, too. The drugs in the tobacco smoke can enter the lungs of the nonsmoker when he or she breathes. Harmful changes also can happen in the nonsmoker's body.

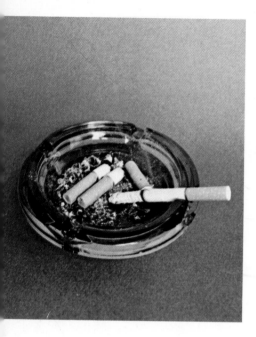

What three substances in tobacco smoke cause changes in a smoker's body?

Tobacco smoke contains many different drugs. All of these drugs act on the body at the same time. Each drug causes a different change in the body. Tobacco smoke makes people feel excited. It also makes people feel weak, tired, and dizzy. All of these changes harm the smoker's health.

The Substances in Tobacco Smoke

One drug in tobacco smoke is **nicotine.** Nicotine makes the openings of the blood vessels smaller than they should be. That makes it hard for the blood to flow easily. Then the heart must work harder to move the blood.

Another drug in tobacco smoke is **tar.** Tar is a sticky, dark brown substance. It coats the inside of the windpipe. Tar in the lungs makes it difficult for oxygen to pass into the smoker's blood. The smoker's cells get less oxygen. The smoker coughs and feels tired.

Tobacco smoke also contains a gas called **carbon monoxide.** Carbon monoxide takes the place of oxygen in a smoker's blood. When the cells cannot get enough oxygen, the smoker feels tired.

How Tobacco Harms People

The drugs in tobacco cause many immediate changes in a smoker's body. The heart beats faster and the smoker feels excited. At the same time, the smoker may feel tired. These changes can happen from smoking only one cigarette.

Tobacco smoke can have very harmful effects on a person's health. Tobacco smoke can tear some of

Thinking About Low Tar Cigarettes

Some cigarettes have less tar than others. They also have less nicotine. Why might cigarette companies make these cigarettes?

the air sacs in the lungs. This is a disease called **emphysema.** People with this disease have a hard time breathing. They run out of breath very easily. There is no cure for emphysema. If people with emphysema keep smoking, they may die.

Sometimes the drugs in tobacco smoke make lumps grow in people's lungs. The lumps make the lungs stop working as they should. This is a disease called **lung cancer.** Many people who get this disease die.

Not all smokers get one of these diseases. But many heavy smokers suffer from poor health. They cough a lot. They run out of breath easily. Many of them live shorter lives than nonsmokers.

Why Do Some People Start Smoking?

Many people know about the dangers of smoking tobacco. But they still smoke. People start smoking for many different reasons. Some people smoke their first cigarette just to see what it is like. Others do it because their friends smoke. Some start smoking to show off. They think smoking makes them look tough or grown-up.

People who smoke do not really look tough. In fact, many smokers are weak and unhealthy. Smoking does not make anyone look more grown-up. But some young people get this idea from movies or from people who smoke. They may get it from advertisements in magazines and newspapers, too. Advertisements often try to give the idea that smoking is a grown-up thing to do. Some people are fooled into believing this idea.

About Cancer

The American Cancer Society reports that the number of cases of lung cancer in women is increasing. The cancer death rate for women who smoke is 67 percent higher than for women who do not smoke.

Looking at Cigarette Advertisements

Look at cigarette advertisements in magazines. What are the people in the ads doing, besides smoking? How do they look? How do they seem to feel? What might be the purpose of these advertisements?

Larry Hagman

Focus On

Larry Hagman, a star of TV's *Dallas,* was successful in breaking a long-term smoking habit. Today, Larry dislikes being near cigarette smoke.

In 1986, Larry was the chairperson of the Great American Smokeout. It was his sixth year in a row as chairperson. The Smokeout was started across the United States in 1977. As chairperson, Larry called for every smoker to stop smoking on the Great American Smokeout day. Smokers are challenged to stop smoking for at least 24 hours. The Smokeout is a great day for many smokers. On that day, they quit smoking for good.

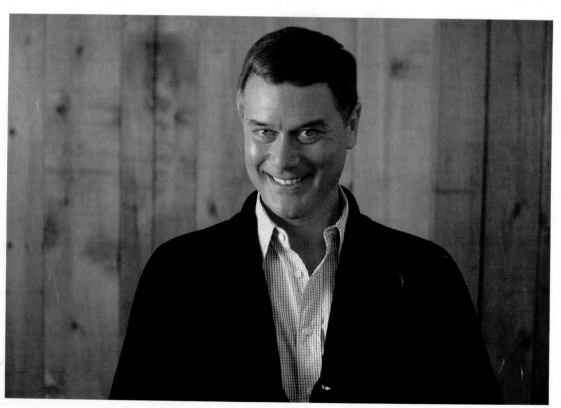

Why Do Some People Keep Smoking?

Many people who smoke wish they had never started. You may wonder why they continue to smoke. The reason is that smoking, especially cigarette smoking, becomes a habit. People who smoke find it very hard to stop even if they want to. Smoking may even make them ill. But every few minutes they want to smoke again.

Scientists do not know why smoking cigarettes becomes a habit. But they know it has something to do with nicotine. Nicotine causes certain changes in a smoker's body. The changes make the smoker want cigarettes all the time. The smoker may form a habit and not know it. When the smoker tries to stop, it may not be easy to do. The smoker may not be able to go without cigarettes for even a few hours.

Breaking the cigarette habit can be very hard. Many smokers try to break their habit and fail. They have to try again and again. It becomes a big problem in their lives. People who do not start smoking never have to face this problem.

Help for Smokers

Smokers who want to stop smoking often can find help. Many hospitals have smoking clinics. Smoking clinics have helped many smokers break the smoking habit.

Wellness Tip

The best time to decide not to smoke is now. Your decision not to smoke will have a positive effect on your wellness.

REVIEW IT NOW

1. How long does it take for tobacco smoke to cause changes in the body?
2. What are three harmful substances in tobacco smoke?
3. What is emphysema?
4. What is lung cancer?
5. What drug in tobacco smoke makes it hard for a person to break the cigarette habit?

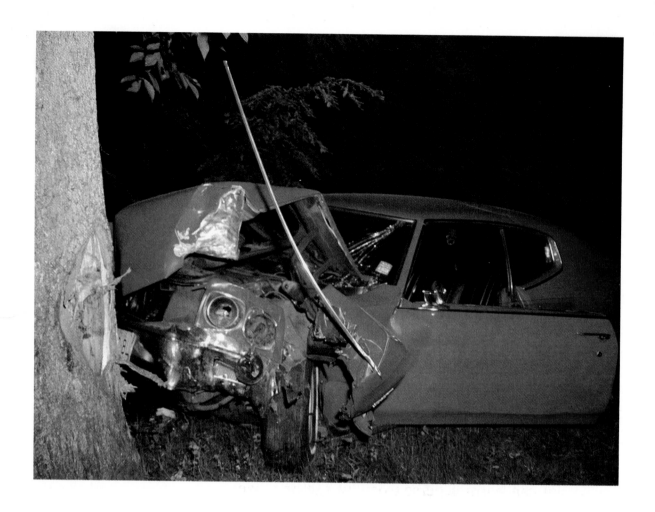

How could a person who has been drinking alcohol prevent this kind of accident?

Alcohol and Personality

Alcohol also can cause changes in a person's personality. This can happen after many years of drinking alcohol. It can even happen after just a few drinks.

ALCOHOL AND YOUR HEALTH

Otis saw some bad news on television. An automobile accident on Old Sawmill Road killed the driver and his passenger. The car had gone off the road and hit a tree. It happened because the driver had been drinking alcohol. The alcohol made him unable to steer the car properly.

Alcohol causes many changes in a person. A little alcohol can change the way a person feels. More alcohol changes how the person acts. Even more alcohol stops the person's body from working properly. Then the person falls asleep and may wake up feeling ill.

How Alcohol Affects the Body

Alcohol slows down the nervous system. The nervous system controls the whole body. Too much alcohol makes people lose control over their bodies. It makes them clumsy and unable to walk in a straight line. The alcohol can make them see everything as a blur. They cannot tell how far away things are. They may crash into things when they try to walk. They can have accidents easily and hurt themselves.

A person must drink a certain amount of alcohol before these changes happen. The amount is different for each person. If you are small, it takes less alcohol to cause changes in your body. And the effects are stronger. The picture helps show that the same amount of alcohol has stronger effects on a small person's body. For a person your age, even a small amount of alcohol can be harmful. A great deal of alcohol can harm a person of any age and size.

Understanding Alcohol and Body Size

Find two glasses of the same size. Fill half of one with water. Fill the other glass full of water. Put one drop of food coloring in each glass. Which changes color more? Which acted more the way your body would act if you drank a small amount of alcohol? Why?

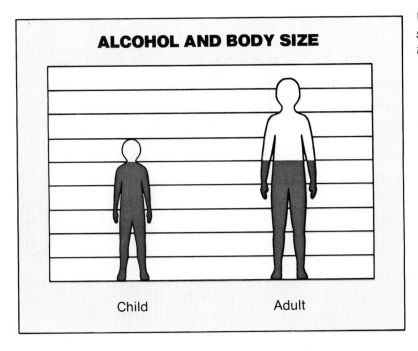

ALCOHOL AND BODY SIZE

Child   Adult

Which person would feel stronger effects if each drank the same amount of alcohol? Why?

What could happen if a person drives a car after drinking a lot of alcohol?

Drinking Alcohol and Driving

Suppose someone drinks a lot of alcohol and then drives a car. The chances are high that the person will have an accident. Alcohol can make people see things as a blur. It can also slow down their actions. They may not see dangers on the road ahead in time to stop. They may turn the wheel too suddenly or drive too fast without knowing it. People may not even know they are making these mistakes after drinking too much alcohol.

People should not drive after they drink alcohol. People who drive after drinking too much alcohol cause many car accidents. Many people are killed in these accidents each year.

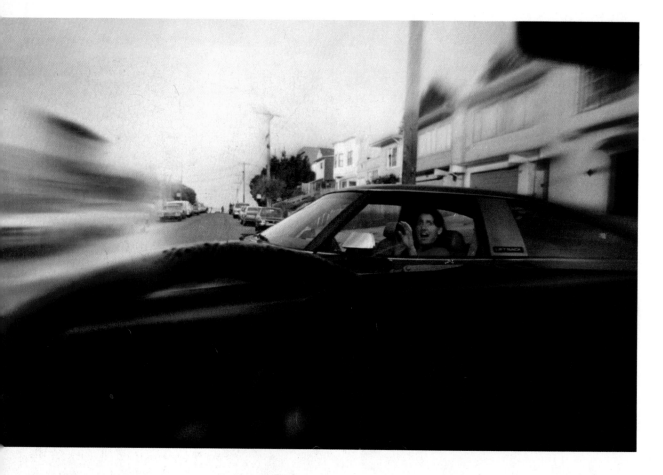

A Breath Test for Alcohol

It is against the law for a person to drive after drinking too much alcohol. But many people do. Police officers can test a person for the amount of alcohol in the blood. They can ask a person to walk in a straight line. Or they can ask a person to take a breath test. They do this with a *breath test machine.*

The breath test machine has a tube connected to it. The person taking the test breathes into the tube. The machine can tell from the amount of alcohol in the breath how much alcohol is in the blood. If the alcohol level in the blood is above a certain limit, the police officer can arrest the person.

Health Today

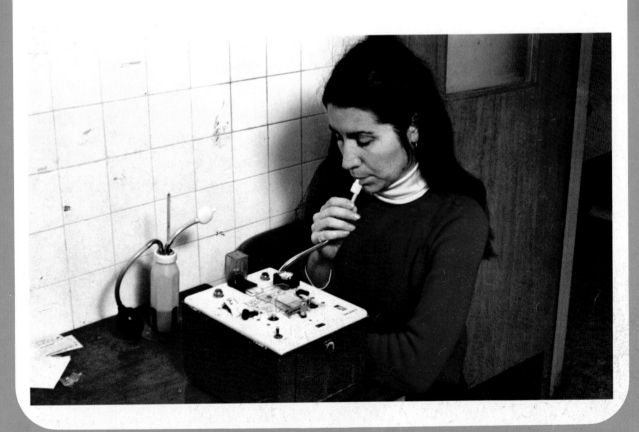

Finding Out About the Effects of Alcohol

Some harmful effects of alcohol are listed on this page. In what other ways can drinking too much alcohol hurt the body?

Helping Alcoholics

Many people realize the dangers of alcohol and alcoholism. Doctors and hospitals often work with alcoholics to help them recover and lead healthful lives.

Other Dangers of Alcohol

Drinking alcohol can become a habit for some people. When they try to stop drinking, they become ill. They need alcohol to feel normal. These people have a disease called **alcoholism.** They are **alcoholics.** Anyone who drinks a lot of alcohol can become an alcoholic. The person can be young or old. Young people who drink alcohol face a greater risk of becoming alcoholics because they have small bodies. Alcohol has very strong effects on them.

Alcoholics seldom can lead normal lives. The alcohol they drink keeps them from doing many things very well. They often lose their jobs or have to leave school. They may lose their friends because of the way alcohol makes them act. Many alcoholics end up in hospitals. But alcoholics can become healthy again if they stop drinking.

Drinking alcohol can harm many parts of the body. It can harm people even if they do not become alcoholics. Alcohol can cause a disease of the liver. It can weaken the heart and harm the brain. It can keep a person from getting enough nutrients. People who drink a lot of alcohol become less and less healthy. They often lead shorter lives than other people.

Why Do Some People Start Using Alcohol?

Some young people see adults drinking beer, wine, or whiskey. They decide that these drinks must be safe. They may not know much about alcohol. Or they may forget that alcohol has strong effects on young people.

They start to wonder what alcohol tastes like. They may decide that drinking alcohol is a grown-up thing to do. For these and other reasons, some young people try drinking alcohol. A few of them drink alcohol again when they have a chance. Some of them even form a habit of drinking.

Sometimes young people talk each other into drinking alcohol. They may try to talk their friends into it by saying that it is fun. They may even dare their friends to drink. They may laugh at them if they refuse. Sometimes their friends give in and take a drink. Sometimes their friends know about alcohol. They refuse the drink.

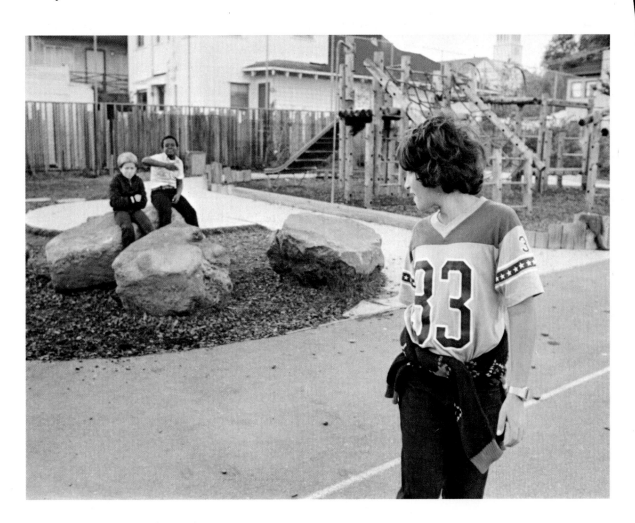

What are some reasons for not drinking alcohol this boy might have given his friends?

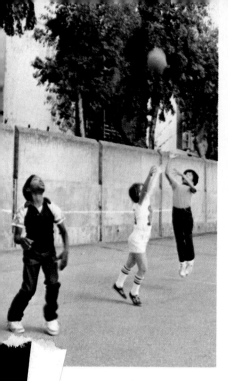
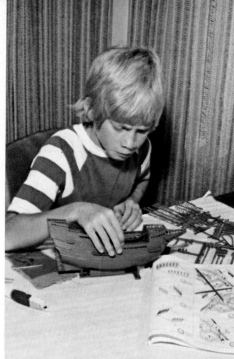
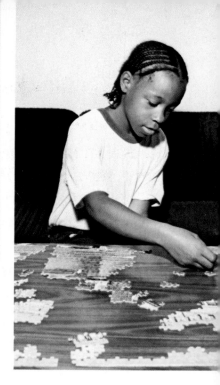

Each of these children is doing something he or she enjoys. In what ways would alcohol make them unable to do these activities?

Avoiding Alcohol

There are many ways to have fun and feel good. Maybe you like to paint or listen to music or play ball. Maybe you like to read or make up funny stories to tell your friends. Drinking alcohol can keep you from enjoying these activities.

The people in these pictures are doing things they enjoy. They would not be able to do these things after drinking alcohol. Each person has at least one reason to avoid alcohol.

REVIEW IT NOW

---

1. What change does alcohol cause in the nervous system?
2. What is alcoholism?
3. What are three parts of the body that can be harmed by drinking alcohol?

Having a Health Council

Have a "health council" with your family. Choose a time when you can meet to talk about safety and drugs. Here are some important questions to answer:

- Are all medicines stored out of the reach of children?
- Are all medicines labeled clearly?
- Are any out of date?
- Do you have a doctor's phone number in case someone takes too much medicine or the wrong medicine by mistake?
- Is this number near the telephone?

By talking about safety and drugs, you and your family can help protect your health.

Working Toward Wellness

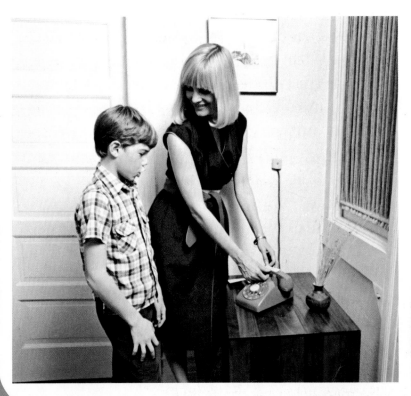

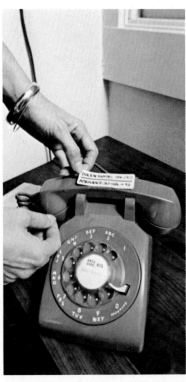

To Help You Review

Checking Your Understanding

Write the numbers from 1 to 13 on your paper. After each number, write the answer to the question or questions. Page numbers in ( ) tell you where to look in the chapter if you need help.

1. What are the unneeded or unneccessary changes in the body caused by a medicine called? **(164)**
2. What is one difference between a prescription medicine and an OTC medicine? **(166–167)**
3. What is caffeine? What does it do to the body? **(169)**
4. How do the drugs in tobacco get to all the cells in a smoker's body? **(171)**
5. What does nicotine do to the body? **(172)**
6. How can the tar in tobacco smoke make a smoker feel tired? **(172)**
7. What are two diseases that smoking cigarettes can cause? **(173)**
8. What are two reasons why some people start smoking? **(173)**
9. Why is it difficult for some people to stop smoking? **(175)**
10. What does alcohol do to the nervous system? **(177)**
11. What may happen to a person who drinks alcohol and then drives a car? **(178)**
12. When a person needs alcohol to feel normal, what disease does he or she have? **(180)**
13. Who can become an alcoholic? **(180)**

Checking Your Health Vocabulary

Write the numbers from 1 to 8 on your paper. After each number, write the letter of the meaning for the word or words. Page numbers in ( ) tell you where to look in the chapter if you need help.

1. drug (**162**)   **5.** alcohol (**170**)
2. medicine (**163**)   **6.** tobacco (**170**)
3. prescription (**166**)   **7.** emphysema (**172–173**)
4. pharmacist (**166**)   **8.** lung cancer (**173**)

a. a specially trained worker who prepares medicines
b. any substance other than food that causes changes in the body
c. a disease caused when tobacco smoke tears air sacs in the lungs
d. a drug that is used to help people who are ill
e. the filling inside cigarettes and cigars that contains drugs
f. a written order from a doctor
g. a disease in which lumps grow inside the lungs
h. a drug found in drinks such as beer and wine

Write the numbers from 9 to 12 on your paper. Then write a sentence that explains the meaning of each word or words. Page numbers in ( ) tell you where to look in the chapter if you need help.

9. prescription medicines (**166**)   **12.** tar (**172**)
10. over-the-counter medicines (**167**)
11. carbon monoxide (**172**)

Practice Test

True or False?

Write the numbers from 1 to 15 on your paper. After each number, write *T* if the sentence is *true*. Write *F* if it is *false*. Rewrite each false sentence to make it true.

1. You should always ask an adult before taking any medicine.
2. A prescription for a medicine is for more than one person.
3. Over-the-counter medicines may have side effects.
4. Some drugs cannot be used as medicines.
5. Drinking coffee slows down a person's heart.
6. It takes less than a minute for tobacco smoke to cause changes in the body.
7. Each drug in tobacco smoke causes a different change in the body.
8. Many heavy smokers live shorter lives than nonsmokers.
9. Emphysema is a serious disease of the heart.
10. It is easy for young people who smoke to break the habit.
11. Only large amounts of alcohol cause changes in the body.
12. It takes only a small amount of alcohol to cause changes in a small person's body.
13. People who drive after drinking cause many car accidents.
14. Only an older person can become an alcoholic.
15. Drinking alcohol can keep a person from getting enough nutrients.

Complete the Sentence

Write the numbers from 16 to 20 on your paper. After each number, copy the sentence and fill in the missing word or words.

16. A drug is any substance other than _____ that causes changes in the body.
17. Every medicine comes with _____ that tell how to use the medicine.
18. Caffeine speeds up the _____ and nerves.
19. Smoking tobacco may cause diseases such as emphysema and _____.
20. Alcohol slows down a person's _____ system.

Learning More

For You to Do

1. Write a letter to the American Cancer Society. Ask for some information about smoking and health. Look in a telephone book for a local address. If your area or a nearby area does not have a local branch, you can write to the American Cancer Society, Vice President for Public Education, 219 East 42nd Street, New York, NY 10017.
2. Call your local police department. Find out about the laws for driving after drinking alcohol. Find out how police can tell if a person is driving after drinking alcohol. What kind of tests do the local police give? What usually happens if the person fails the test? Share your information with your class.

For You to Find Out

1. What does a *pharmacist* do? For how many years must a person go to school in order to be a pharmacist? Books on careers might have the information. You also might ask a pharmacist to answer your questions.

2. About how many people who get lung cancer each year are smokers? The American Cancer Society or the American Lung Association might have this information. Look in a telephone book for the phone number of a local branch of each group.
3. What are generic OTC medicines? How are they different from OTC medicines made popular by TV and magazine ads? You might ask a pharmacist to tell you about generic medicines.

For You to Read

Here are some books you can look for in your school or public library to find out more about drugs.

Madison, Arnold. *Drugs and You.* Messner, 1982

Seixas, Judith S. *Tobacco: What It Is, What It Does.* Greenwillow, 1981.

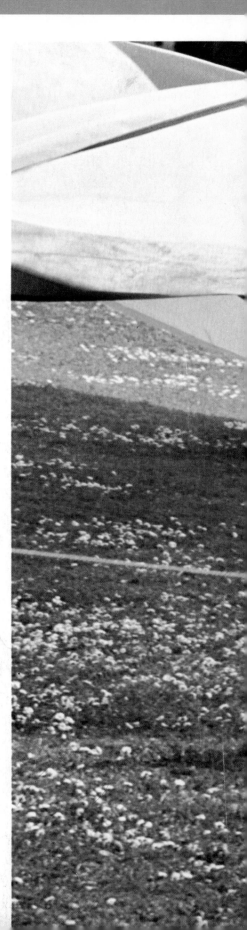

CHAPTER 8

Keeping Safe

Accidents can happen at any time and at any place. They can happen when you are playing. They can happen at home or at school. Sometimes they happen for no reason. Other times they happen because someone was not careful.

Accidents are one of the greatest dangers to your wellness. Knowing how accidents happen may help you prevent many of them. You can be aware of dangers that may cause accidents. You can plan ahead for safety. Being careful is the best self-defense you can have against accidents.

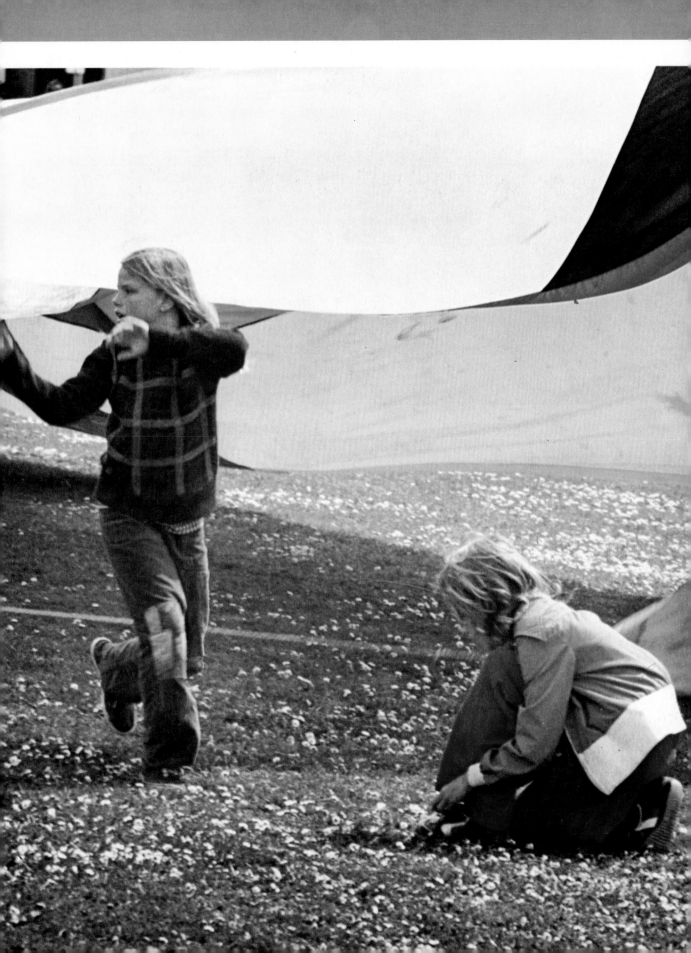

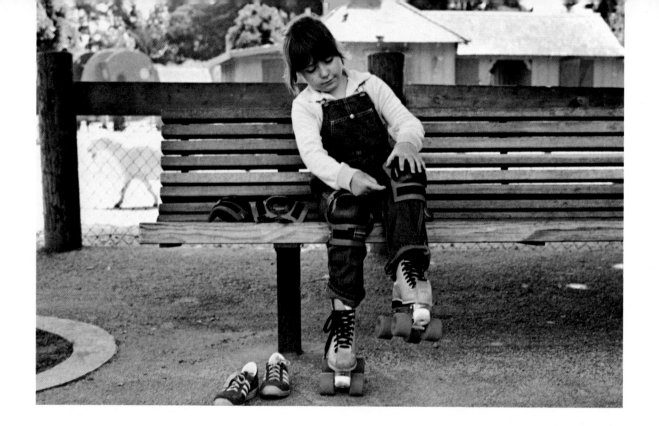

How is this girl helping to keep herself safe?

PLANNING AHEAD FOR SAFETY

You can do many things to keep yourself healthy. You can eat healthful foods. You can get regular exercise and enough sleep. You can keep yourself clean.

Sometimes doing things to take care of your health is not enough. Your health could be harmed by an unexpected event. Such an unexpected event is called an **accident.**

Accidents happen even when you think ahead and follow safety rules. You should know what to do when an accident happens. Knowing what to do could save someone's life.

You can learn when and where many accidents happen. You can find out how to have fewer accidents. And you can learn what to do in case an accident does happen. Then you can plan ahead for safety.

Accidental Death

More than 100,000 deaths in the United States each year are caused by accidents. Most of the accidents that cause death are motor vehicle accidents, falls, drownings, fires and burns, and poisonings.

When and Where Accidents Can Happen

Tom walks to and from school every day. On his way he passes a softball field. One afternoon, as Tom was walking by, a player hit a foul ball. The ball hit Tom on the arm and caused a bruise.

Tom's injury was an accident. It could have happened to anyone walking by the field. It also could have happened at any time when people were playing softball.

Accidents can happen anywhere, to anyone, and at almost any time. You can have an accident outside, at school, or in your home. You can have an accident while you are playing or while you are working. No one can be completely safe from accidents.

Why was Tom's injury an accident?

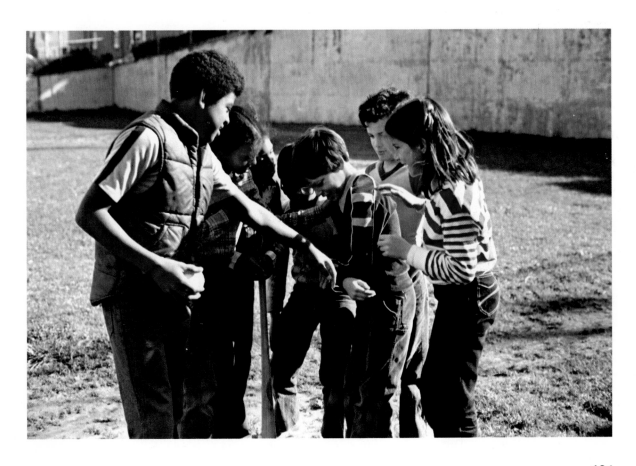

How Accidents Can Be Avoided

Ms. Harris's class was discussing accidents and safety. The students made a chart showing the kinds of accidents each of them had during the past week.

The class talked about how many accidents each student had had. During the week, Bruce and Marcia had the most accidents. Jonathan had the fewest. Ms. Harris found out that Jonathan was careful and followed safety rules.

You can avoid many accidents by being aware of safety. If you think ahead and follow safety rules, you will probably have fewer accidents.

Look at the chart that Ms. Harris's class made. Why might Jonathan have had the fewest accidents?

ACCIDENTS THIS WEEK

	Bicycling	Roller-skating	Tripped While Running	Swimming	Sunburn	Almost Run Over While Walking
Kristin	X				X	
Ben		X				X
Jonathan			X			
Rita	X	X				
Marcia	X	X	X			X
Bruce	X			X	X	X
Kim		X	X			
Margo	X					X

Acting in an Emergency

Many accidents happen even when people think ahead and follow safety rules. Sometimes an accident is serious and help is needed right away. It is an **emergency.** Car accidents and fires are emergencies that happen often.

When there is an emergency, you must stay calm. If you do not stay calm, you may not be able to think clearly. You may not know what to do.

In an emergency, you must think fast and decide what to do. You may need an adult to help you. You should know whom to call for help. A doctor may be needed. The police or fire department may have to be called. And you may have to act on your own until help arrives. By thinking clearly and knowing whom to call for help, you can help keep yourself and others safe.

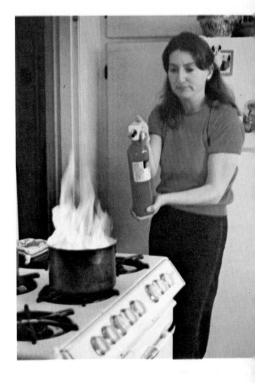

Why is it important to stay calm in an emergency?

REVIEW IT NOW

1. What is an accident?
2. What can you do to avoid accidents?
3. What is an emergency?
4. What should you do in an emergency?

Focus On

Freddie Bell

Two North Carolina women and their seven cats may be alive today because of Freddie Bell. Early one December morning in 1980, Freddie left his home to go to work. He saw smoke coming from a nearby house. Freddie called the fire department and then ran across the street. He started knocking on the door and yelling to the people inside.

Freddie knew what to do in an emergency. First, he reported the emergency. Then he alerted the people in the house. He did not enter the burning building.

Freddie's story was in the *Wilmington Morning Star.* And his job? He delivers that same newspaper!

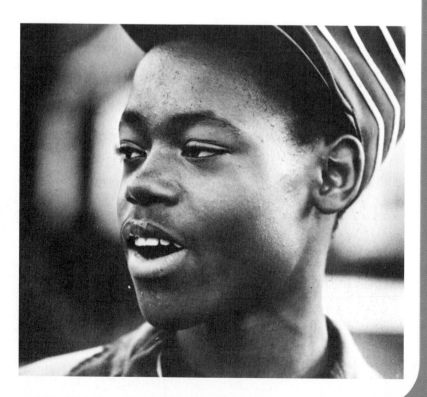

BICYCLE SAFETY

Children your age have more bicycle accidents than any other kind of accident. You need to watch for many things when riding a bicycle. You have to watch for cars and traffic signals. You have to watch for holes in the street. You also have to watch for people who are walking and for other bicycle riders.

You can avoid most bicycle accidents by following safety rules and making sure that car drivers can see you.

Riding Safely

Kristin and Ben enjoy riding their bicycles to school. But they do not ride side by side. Kristin and Ben ride single file. They ride close to the right-hand curb. They always ride in the same direction as traffic.

In what ways are Kristin and Ben riding safely?

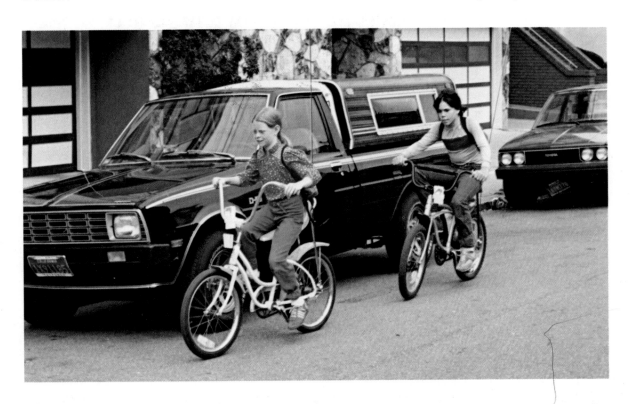

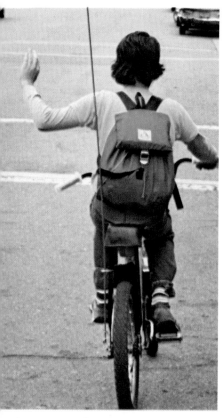
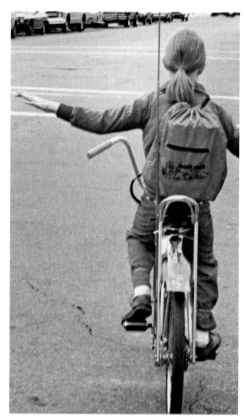
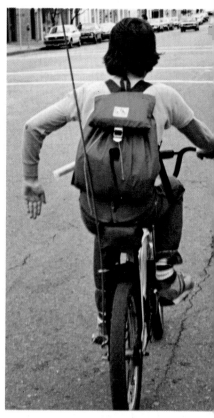

| right turn | left turn | stop |

Look at the pictures of hand signals for a right turn, a left turn, and a stop. Practice these hand signals with a friend.

Using Bicycle Paths

You can ride more safely if you ride your bicycle on bike paths. Not all bike paths are along the sides of streets. Some are in parks. Watch for signs that tell you where bike paths or routes are.

Ben and Kristin carry their books in a basket or knapsack—not in their hands. They can keep both hands on the handlebars when they are riding. The only time they take one of their hands off the handlebars is to signal. They want car drivers to know when they are about to turn or stop. The pictures show the signals they use.

When Ben and Kristin ride their bicycles, they stay alert. They ride slowly if the street is rough or wet. They slow down every time they approach a crossing. They walk their bicycles across streets, using the crosswalk. They watch for cars starting out from the curb or from a driveway. They also watch for people opening car doors. People in cars may not see someone on a bicycle.

Making Sure Others See You

Kristin and Ben use hand signals so that car drivers will see them and know when they are about to turn. They have made their bicycles more visible to drivers, too. They have put flags on their bicycles so people can see them during the daytime. For riding at night, each of them has a lamp on the handlebars. Each also has a white or yellow reflector on the bicycle's front and back wheels. They also have reflectors on the backs of their pedals. When Ben and Kristin ride, they wear bright-colored clothing so drivers can see them.

By being aware of bicycle safety, you can avoid many accidents. Remember to follow all bicycle safety rules. Be careful and alert whenever you ride your bicycle. Make sure that your bicycle is working properly. Be sure that other people can see you when you are on your bicycle. When you follow all these rules, bicycle riding can be safe and fun.

What has Ben put on his bicycle for safety?

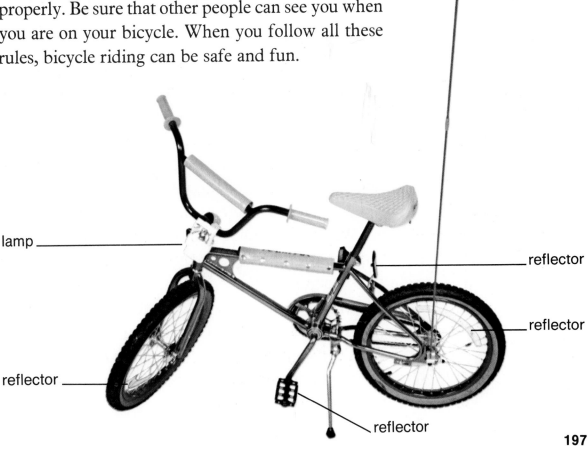

flag

lamp

reflector

reflector

reflector

reflector

197

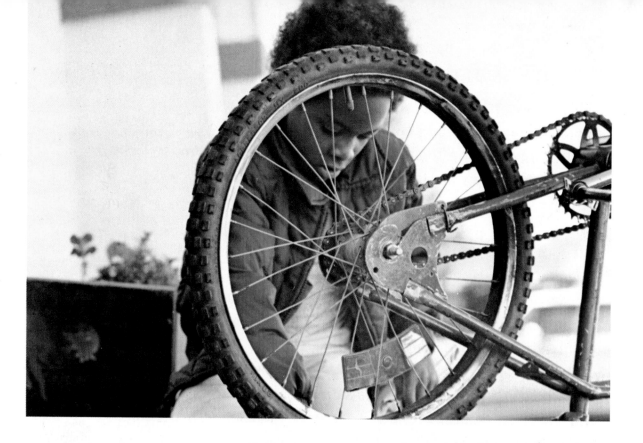

How can keeping your bicycle in good working order help you keep safe?

Bicycle Safety Rules
• Always stay alert.   • Obey all traffic rules, lights, and signs.   • Always ride single file.   • Always ride in the same direction as traffic.   • Do not carry another person on your bicycle.   • Always ride a bicycle that is the right size for you.   • Do not do stunts when you ride a bicycle.   • Keep your bicycle in good working order.

REVIEW IT NOW

1. Where on the street should a person ride a bicycle?
2. Why should a bicycle rider use hand signals?
3. What are three bicycle safety rules for riding at night?

PEDESTRIAN SAFETY

Many people have accidents while walking. A person who is walking is a **pedestrian.** Pedestrians who walk near traffic are often in danger because drivers may not see them. Pedestrians should stay out of the way of cars and always should watch for them.

Jonathan and Rita walk to school together every day. They choose a route that has sidewalks for most of the way. They stay on the sidewalks except to cross a street.

When Rita and Jonathan come to the part of their route that has no sidewalk, they walk close to the edge of the street. They stay on the left-hand side of the street so that they can see oncoming traffic. They walk single file.

Jonathan and Rita are careful never to break traffic rules. They do not walk or run into a street from between parked cars. They cross streets only at corners or crosswalks. They obey traffic signals. They cross the street only when they have a green light or a WALK signal. They also obey directions from police officers or crossing guards.

Which pedestrian safety rules are Rita and Jonathan following?

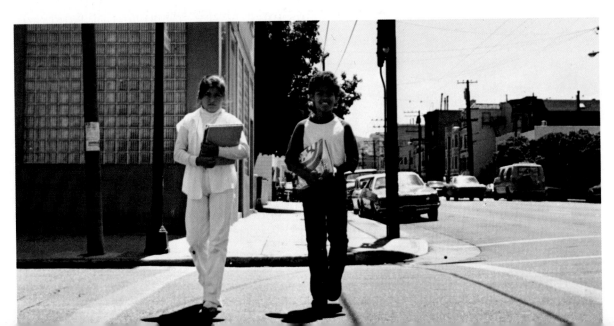

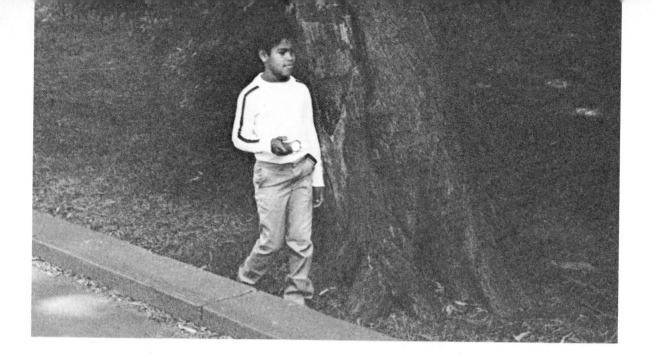

How is Jonathan keeping safe as he walks in the early evening?

As a pedestrian, you should always be alert for cars. When you come to a crossing, look both ways. Watch for cars that are turning, too. Wait on the curb for cars to pass or for the light to change. Be sure that all cars have stopped before you step into the street. As you cross, continue to watch for cars. Be sure the drivers see you.

If you walk at night, wear bright-colored clothing so that drivers will see you. Carry a flashlight if you walk where there are no bright street lights.

Pedestrians must always be aware of safety. If you stay alert and obey all traffic rules, you will have fewer accidents while walking.

REVIEW IT NOW

1. What is a pedestrian?
2. What should a pedestrian always be alert for?
3. What should a pedestrian do at night?

Police Officer

An empty building, speeding traffic, or an unsafe bicycle—all can mean a threat to safety. But the *police officer* is trained to protect the public from such dangers.

Police officers help make the public aware of safety. Some police officers give advice about home safety. Often, police officers visit schools to talk to students about bicycle safety.

A person with a high school diploma can train to be a police officer. To learn more about police work and training, write to the International Association of Chiefs of Police, 13 Firstfield Road, P.O. Box 6010, Gaithersburg, MD 20878.

Health Career

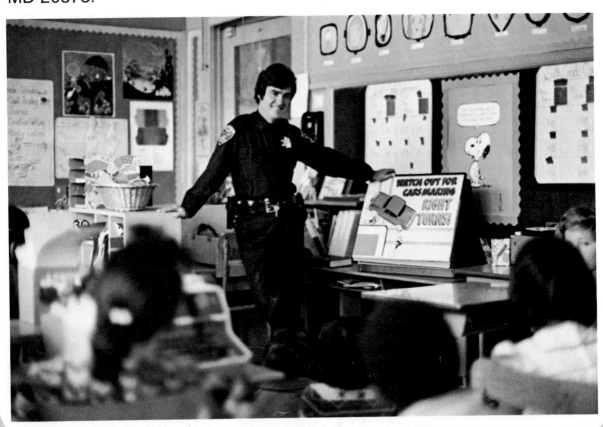

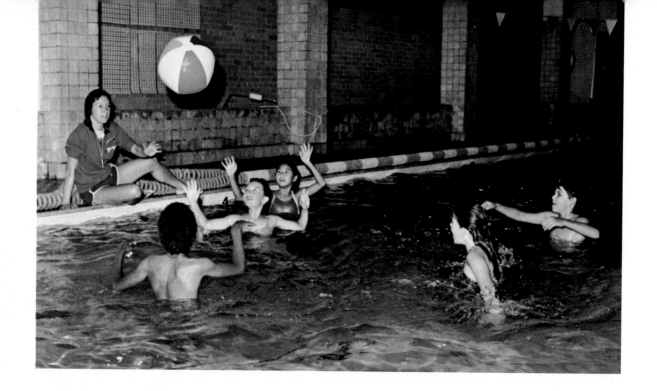

Why should you wait to swim until the lifeguard is on duty?

SAFETY NEAR WATER

Many accidents happen in or near water. Many people who drown have fallen into the water by accident. Even good swimmers can have trouble in the water if they get tired or if the water is too rough or too cold. You always should be aware of safety when you are playing near water.

Safety in Swimming

Margo climbed out of the swimming pool and walked to the dressing room. She was late for dinner, but she did not run. She knew it was not safe to run next to the swimming pool. The pavement could be wet and slippery. She could fall on the pavement or into the pool. By thinking about safety, Margo avoided an accident.

Bruce and Kim came to the pool early one day. The lifeguard was not on duty yet. Bruce wanted to

Swimming Safely

It can be dangerous to swim for too long in cold water. Cold water lowers body temperature. Normal body temperature is 98.6°F (36°C). The first sign of lowered body temperature is shivering. If you begin to shiver while you are swimming, get out of the water.

jump into the water. Kim said that they should wait for the lifeguard. If they had trouble before the lifeguard came, nobody would be there to help them.

Later Bruce thought it would be fun to pretend that he was drowning. Kim talked him out of it. She said that someone else might really need help at the same time. And if Bruce had trouble later, the lifeguard might think he was still pretending.

Being aware of safety is important when you go swimming. Make sure that you never swim alone. If you needed help, the lifeguard might not see you, and no one would be with you to call for help. If possible, have an adult who swims well nearby when you are swimming.

Many places have special rules for swimmers. These rules are usually posted on a sign near the water. Obey any signs you see when you go swimming.

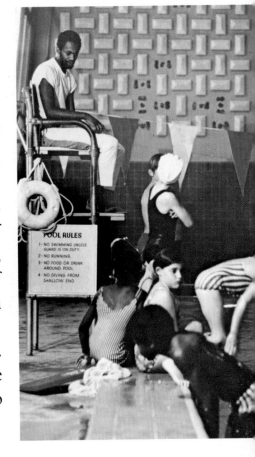

Why should you read the swimming safety rules before you swim?

Other Places to Swim

People do not always swim in swimming pools. They also swim in lakes, streams, rivers, and oceans. All these places have special safety rules.

- Swim only in areas that you know are safe. Do not swim where the waves are high or where the current is strong.
- Always find out how deep the water is before you jump in.
- Never swim farther than you know you can. It is difficult to tell how far it is across a lake or river.
- Always stay close to shore so you can swim to safety if you become tired.
- Check the area where you are going to swim for rocks, tree branches, or other hidden objects that could harm you.

Safety in Boating

Last summer Kristin, Ben, Jonathan, Rita, and their families camped near a lake. Kristin's father took the children out in a boat one day. Everyone put on a life jacket before getting into the boat. If the boat tipped over, the life jackets would help them float.

In the boat, everyone was careful to sit still. If one person had moved around too much or stood up, the boat might have tipped over.

You should never get into a boat without an adult. If an accident happens, the adult can help you. Always wear a life jacket in a boat, even when the water is calm and not very deep.

Many accidents can happen while boating. You could fall out of the boat. The boat could run into something. It could leak or turn over.

A boat that turns over can still float upside-down. Hold on to the boat to stay afloat. If you stay with the boat, it will be easier for someone to see you and to rescue you.

Why is it important to wear a life jacket while boating?

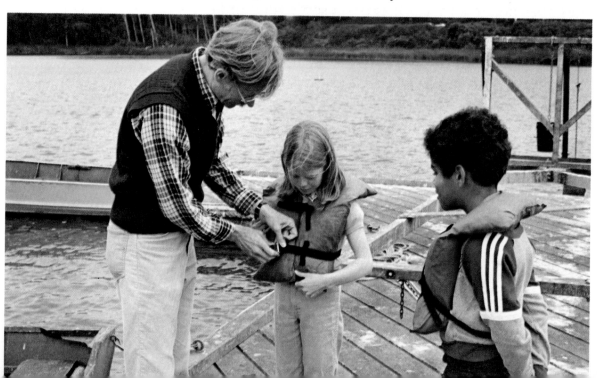

If you are going boating, tell someone who is not going where you plan to go and when you plan to be back. That person may be able to help if you have any trouble.

Helping Someone in Trouble

Rita stayed in the water too long one day. She became tired and called for help. The lifeguard began rowing toward her in his boat. Kristin was on the dock. She threw a life preserver to Rita. Rita held on to it so she could stay afloat until the lifeguard reached her.

Kristin did not jump into the water to help Rita. Kristin had not taken a lifesaving course. She knew that she could not help Rita by herself. If Rita were frightened, she might pull Kristin under the water. Both girls could drown.

If you see someone in trouble in the water, call loudly for help. Do not jump into the water to save the person. Instead, reach out with a towel, a pole, or a branch. If the person is far away, throw a life preserver tied to a rope. Hold on to something or lie on your stomach so that you will not be pulled into the water. When the person grabs what you have reached out or thrown, pull him or her to safety. If you do not have a life preserver, throw anything that floats. Then the person can hold on to it and keep floating until help arrives.

Playing in or near water is fun when you know how to avoid accidents. To stay safe, learn how to swim or float. Remember water safety rules. If you think ahead and watch out for possible dangers, you can help prevent accidents.

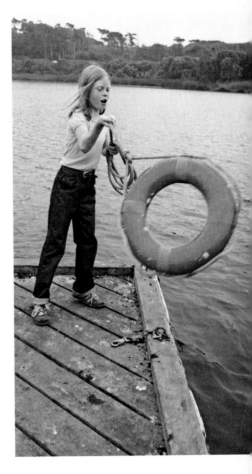

What is Kristin doing to help her friend who is in trouble in the water?

Finding Out About Swimming Courses

What swimming courses are given in your city or town? Are there any courses for beginners? Where and when are beginner courses given?

Survival Floating

If you get into trouble while you are in the water, follow these rules for survival floating.

- Stay calm. Do not thrash about or try to hold your head above water all the time.
- Take a deep breath. Relax. Let yourself sink. Move your arms and legs slowly. You will stay near the surface of the water.
- When you let out the air, lift your head above water. Take a breath.

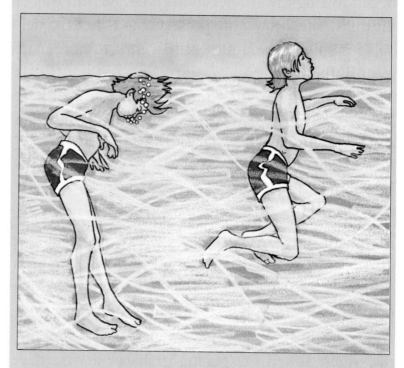

- Relax and repeat these steps until help arrives.

REVIEW IT NOW

1. When are three times good swimmers might have trouble?
2. Why should you never swim alone?
3. What is a life jacket for?
4. What is a life preserver for?

American Red Cross Safety Courses

Health Today

Your community may have several groups, such as the American Red Cross, that give safety courses. One of the courses given by the American Red Cross is especially for people your age.

Basic Aid Training, called *BAT,* teaches you ways to prevent accidents. It helps you to be prepared in case an accident does happen. It teaches you how to handle some common emergencies, too. BAT can teach you what to do if a person is bleeding or is burned.

The American Red Cross also gives other safety courses. These courses are for people of any age who want to learn how to keep safe.

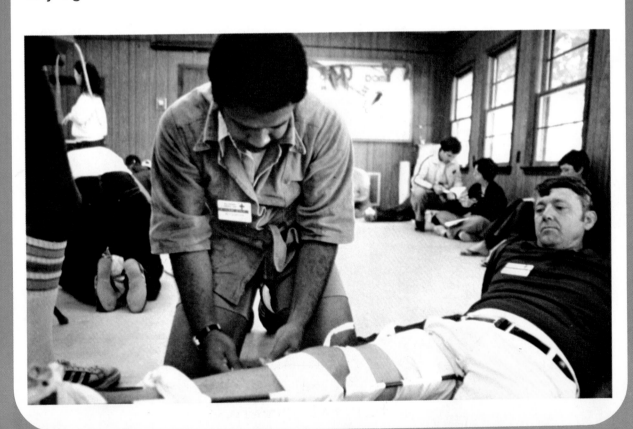

SAFETY AT PLAY

Most people know that accidents can happen while they are riding a bicycle or swimming in a lake. But they may not be thinking about safety when they are playing. Remember that accidents can happen anywhere and at any time.

Choosing Safe Places to Play

Bruce and Marcia wanted to play hide-and-seek in the empty building near their school. Bruce thought the building would have plenty of hiding places. Kristin suggested that they play at her house instead. She did not think the building was a safe place to play. Kristin saw the broken windows and knew there was a lot of glass lying around.

Some places are not safe for playing. Streets and parking lots are made for cars and bicycles, not playing. Building sites could have hidden holes, loose boards, or dangerous tools. You could trip over

What makes this building unsafe for play?

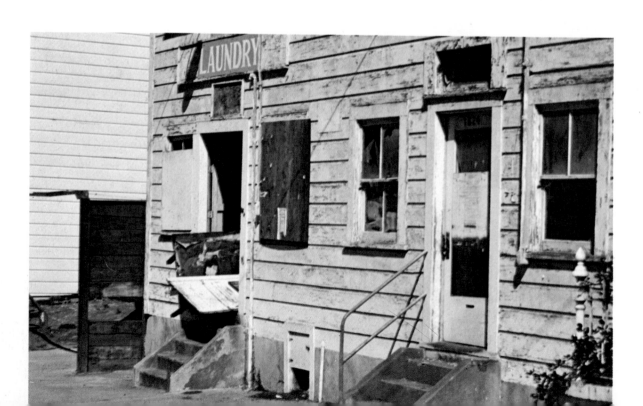

these objects and fall. You could step on a nail or other sharp object. Junkyards are full of broken machinery. You could cut yourself on sharp edges or get trapped inside something like an old refrigerator. Playing near railroad tracks is dangerous, too. You might get hit by a train. You can avoid many accidents by choosing a safe place to play.

Playing Near Home

Jonathan is learning to roller-skate. He practices on the sidewalk in front of his house. He tries to keep from hurting himself by wearing pads on his knees and elbows. He does not try any stunts. He looks out for people on the sidewalk and for cars in driveways.

Even near your home or school there are dangers. Before you start any active games in your own yard, check for hoses or tools that you could trip over. In a playground, make sure that the equipment is not wet before you climb on it. Wet equipment is slippery, and you could fall.

How does Jonathan keep safe while he roller-skates?

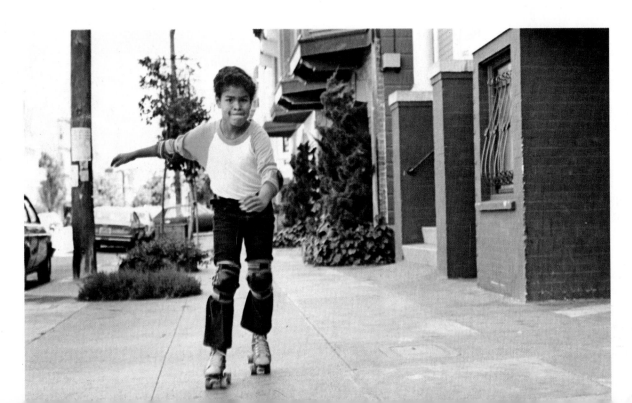

What should Bruce do to protect his skin while lying in the sun?

Playing in the Sun

Bruce likes to be outside in the summer. He likes to lie in the sun to get tanned. He knows he could get a bad sunburn if he stayed in the sun too long. He knows that sunburn often can make a person ill. At the beginning of the summer, Bruce spent only a few minutes in the sun every day. Each day he stayed out a little longer until he was used to being in the sun for an hour or two.

While Bruce is lying in the sun, he uses a suntan lotion that blocks out the sun's most harmful rays. The lotion protects his skin. Bruce does not lie out in the sun in the early afternoon. The sun's rays are strongest and most harmful at that time of day. And he is careful not to go to sleep. Being careful in all these ways helps Bruce prevent a sunburn.

Being in the sunshine feels good, but you must be careful not to stay out too long. That way you can keep from getting sunburned.

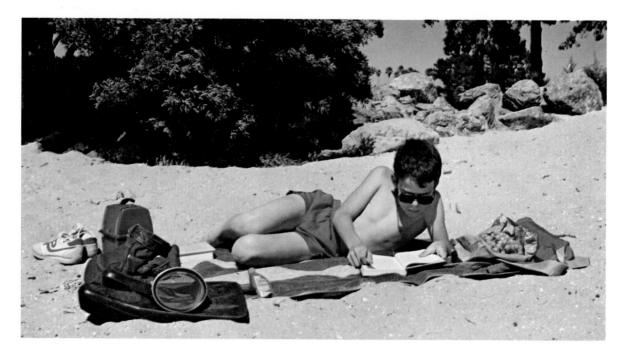

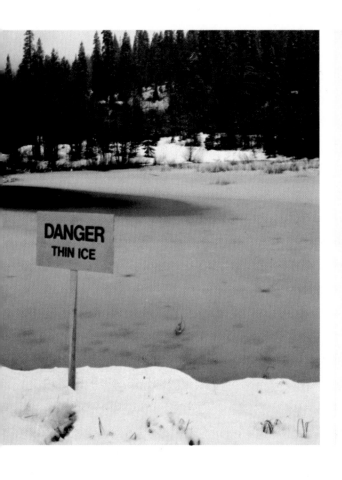

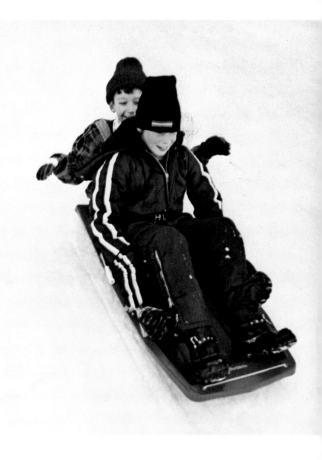

What are two important safety rules to follow when ice-skating or sledding in the winter?

During the winter, Bruce likes to play outdoors. He likes to ice-skate and go sledding. He skates only on ponds or lakes where areas are marked off for skating. There the ice is thick enough to be safe. When Bruce goes sledding, he chooses a hill that has no trees to run into. He also stays away from roads so that he will not slide into a car's path.

Bruce dresses in warm clothes when he goes outdoors to play in the winter. You should dress warmly, too. If you get cold, you could become ill. Always wear a hat, gloves, and something warm on your feet. If you do not, your body will lose much of its warmth. By dressing warmly in the winter, you can stay healthy and have fun, too.

Finding Out About Frostbite

What is **frostbite**? How do people get frostbitten? What can you do to keep from getting frostbite when you play in the cold? Health books in the library may help you find out.

Playing on Holidays

Playing on holidays can be fun, but there are special dangers to watch out for.

Ben and his family went on a Fourth of July picnic. Many people in the park were using firecrackers. But Ben's family knew that people could be badly hurt by them. They stayed away from people who were using them.

On Halloween, Jonathan made a scary costume. It was brightly colored so that people could see him. He did not wear a mask because masks are hard to see through. So he painted on a scary face with makeup instead.

Jonathan and Rita went trick-or-treating together. They made sure their treats would be safe. They stayed in their own neighborhood. Then they went to Rita's house for cider. Before eating any of their treats, they let Rita's mother look at them.

Some special days bring extra danger. To have a good time without being hurt on a holiday, you should think about the dangers. That will help you avoid accidents and have fun.

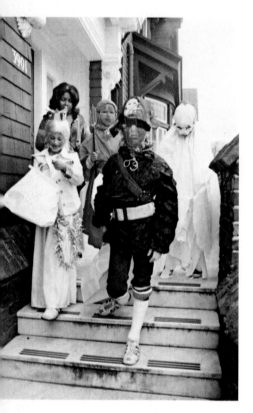

Why is it important to think ahead about dangers on a holiday?

REVIEW IT NOW

1. Where are five places that may not be safe for playing?
2. How can playing in the sun be dangerous?
3. What are three special holiday dangers to watch out for?

Making a Safety Poster

You and your family or friends can become more aware of safety. Make a safety poster for an activity you enjoy.

Choose one of your favorite activities. Here is a list of activities that may help you.

- bicycling
- swimming
- skateboarding
- ice skating

- fishing
- hiking
- roller skating
- camping

Make a safety poster for your activity. Write a catchy saying or slogan that tells an important safety rule. Use your own drawings or cut pictures from magazines that help show your safety rule. You may want to hang your poster at home or at school.

Working Toward Wellness

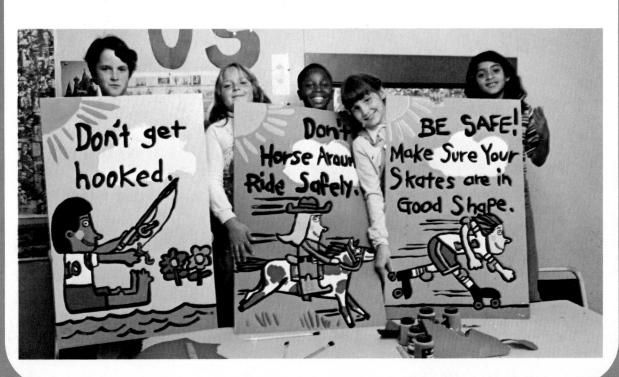

To Help You Review

Checking Your Understanding

Write the numbers from 1 to 13 on your paper. After each number, write the answer to the question or questions. Page numbers in ( ) tell you where to look in the chapter if you need help.

1. Why is it important to know what to do if an accident happens? (**190**)
2. When and where do accidents happen? (**191**)
3. Why must you stay calm in an emergency? (**193**)
4. What are five things to watch for when riding a bicycle? (**195**)
5. What are five things that should be on a bicycle for safety? (**197**)
6. What are four rules pedestrians should follow when crossing a street? (**199–200**)
7. When can even good swimmers have trouble in the water? (**202**)
8. When should you wear a life jacket in a boat? Why? (**204**)
9. If you are going boating, why should you tell your plans to someone who is not going? (**205**)
10. What should you do first if you see someone in trouble in the water? (**205**)
11. What are three ways you can protect yourself from sunburn? (**210**)
12. Why is it important to dress warmly in the winter? (**211**)
13. What are two safety rules to follow if you go trick-or-treating on Halloween? (**212**)

Checking Your Health Vocabulary

Write the numbers from 1 to 3 on your paper. After each number, write the letter of the meaning for the word. Page numbers in ( ) tell you where to look in the chapter if you need help.

1. accident (**190**)
2. emergency (**193**)
3. pedestrian (**199**)

a. a serious accident for which help is needed right away
b. an unexpected event that can harm a person's health
c. a person who is walking

Write the numbers from 4 to 6 on your paper. After each number, write whether the picture shows a *left turn* signal, a *right turn* signal, or a *stop* signal.

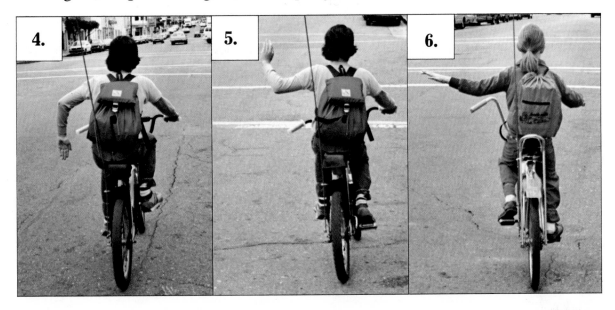

Practice Test

True or False?

Write the numbers from 1 to 15 on your paper. After each number, write *T* if the sentence is *true*. Write *F* if it is *false*. Rewrite each false sentence to make it true.

1. Accidents never happen if you follow safety rules.
2. Knowing what to do in an emergency can save lives.
3. Staying calm in an emergency can help you think clearly.
4. Always ride your bicycle on the left-hand side of the street, facing traffic.
5. Always ride your bicycle across the street, using the crosswalk.
6. Car drivers often do not see pedestrians.
7. If the light is green, you do not need to watch for cars as you cross the street.
8. Wearing bright-colored clothing can help you be safe when you walk at night.
9. Even a good swimmer can have trouble in water that is too rough or too cold.
10. It is safe to swim alone if a lifeguard is on duty.
11. You do not need to wear a life jacket in a boat if the water is calm and not very deep.
12. You should not jump into the water to help someone in trouble.
13. Learning how to swim or float can help you stay safe.
14. You should check your own yard for dangers before you play.
15. Halloween masks can be unsafe to wear because they often are hard to see through.

Complete the Sentence

Write the numbers from 16 to 20 on your paper. After each number, copy the sentence and fill in the missing word or words.

16. Bicycle riders should use _____ _____ to show when they are about to stop or turn.
17. Bicycles should have _____ on their wheels and pedals.
18. Pedestrians should always watch for _____.
19. If someone is in trouble in the water, throw something that _____ to the person.
20. You can avoid many _____ by choosing safe places to play.

Learning More

For You to Do

1. Make a chart like the one Ms. Harris's class made. (See page 192.) Show all the accidents you have had in the past two weeks. Could any of them have been avoided? How?

2. Make a street map of your home or school neighborhood. Put a blue dot by each intersection (place where two streets cross) that has a crosswalk. Put a red dot by each intersection that has a traffic light. Put a yellow dot by each intersection that has stop signs on both streets. Which intersections might be the safest for a pedestrian or bike rider to cross?

For You to Find Out

1. What kinds of accidents happen most often to people your age? How can these accidents be kept from happening so often? You might talk to an ambulance worker or someone who works in the emergency room of a hospital.

2. Does your city or town have bicycle lanes? Where are they located? To find out, call your local public works department or the department of transportation.

3. What is *mouth-to-mouth breathing?* When might a person need mouth-to-mouth breathing? How is it given? Books about first aid can help you find out.

For You to Read

Here are some books you can look for in your school or public library to find out more about safety.

Brown, Marc, and Krensky, Stephen. *Dinosaurs Beware! A Safety Guide.* Atlantic Monthly Press Books, 1982.

Chlad, Dorothy. *Riding on a Bus.* Children's Press, 1985.

Schlachter, Rita. *Good Luck, Bad Luck.* Troll Associates, 1986.

Stone, Judith. *Minutes to Live.* Raintree Publishers, 1980.

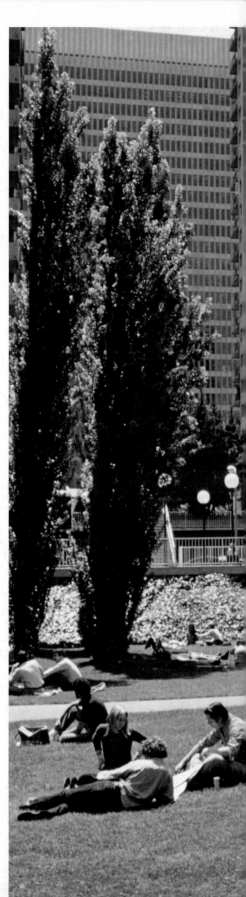

CHAPTER 9

Living in a Healthful Environment

Everyone needs a healthy and safe place to live. Towns and cities have laws to keep them healthy and safe. There are people where you live who work to protect your health and safety.

Some towns and cities have health problems caused by the people who live there. Dirty air and water are two problems that many cities have. Even too much noise can be a health problem.

Some of these problems can be solved by people working together. You can help, too. You can help yourself reach wellness by helping to make your community a healthful place to live.

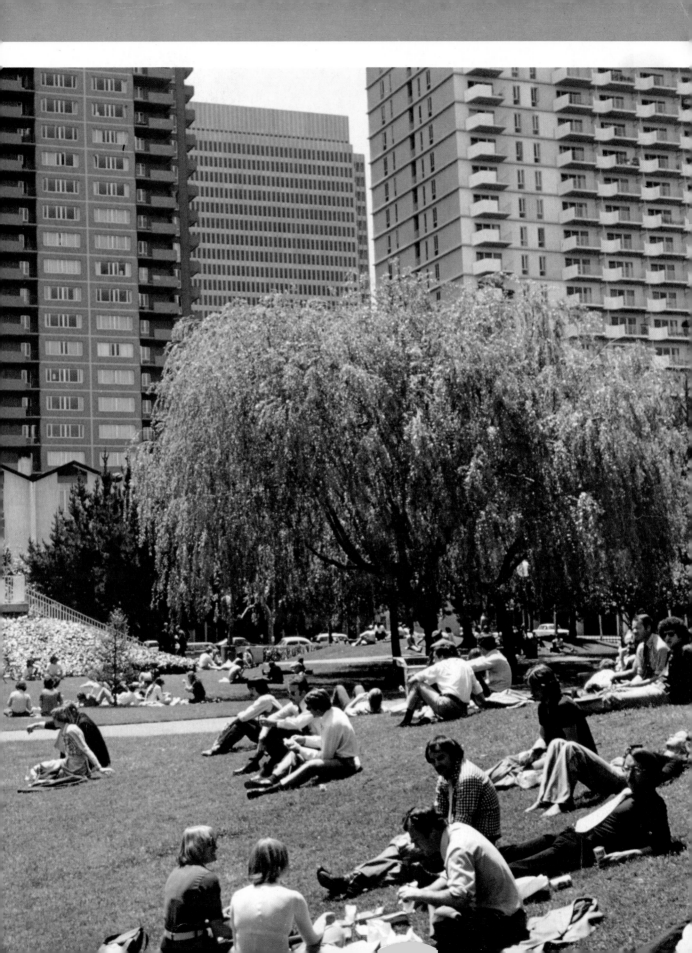

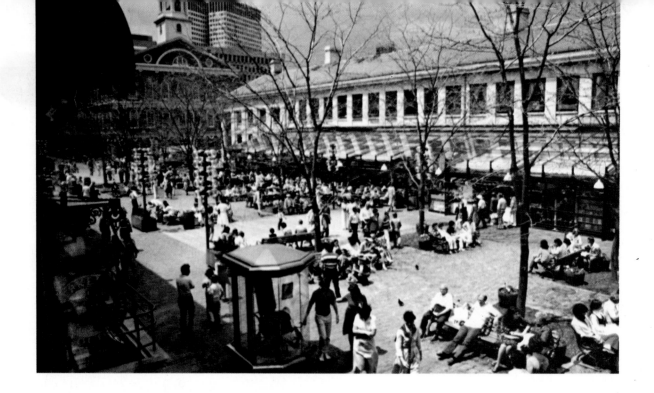

What things do the people in a community depend on?

MAKING YOUR COMMUNITY HEALTHY AND SAFE

A **community** is a group of people who depend on one another. They all depend on the earth's air, water, and land to stay alive. Usually they live in the same place. A community may be very small or very large. It can be one family or all the families living on one street. All the people living on the earth are a community.

The people in a community depend on the same **environment.** The environment is everything in and around the community. It includes all the nonliving things, such as air, water, and soil. It also includes all the living things, such as the people, animals, and plants.

Most people in the community work for health and safety in different ways. Some people in each community are special helpers. Their job is working to keep other people healthy and safe.

Thinking About Communities

There are many kinds of communities. List all of the communities in which you live. How do the people in your communities depend on one another?

220

Health Workers

Some of the special helpers in a community work to prevent disease. These people are **health workers.** They make sure that the food and water are clean and safe for people to use. They take care of the health of the people and animals in the community.

Spoiled food can be a danger to a person's wellness. Food must be inspected, or checked, to make sure it is free of harmful microbes.

Ms. Saito is a food inspector. She makes sure that harmful microbes do not get into the food that people eat. She works in places where food is handled. She visits restaurants and goes to factories and stores where food is prepared. She checks to see that the kitchen or factory is clean. She checks food that is put into cans. She also looks at the food that will be sold in markets. She makes sure that the food is safe to eat.

Finding Out About Community Workers

What kinds of community workers does your community have? How do these workers help keep your community healthy and safe?

In what ways do health workers help prevent disease?

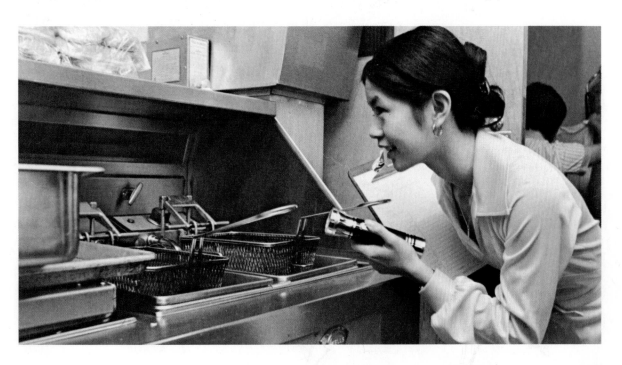

Thinking About Water Testing

What might happen if the drinking water in your community were never tested?

Unclean water can also be a danger to people's wellness. A community's drinking water must be checked to see if it is safe to drink.

Ms. Garcia's job is to inspect the water in her community. She takes samples of the drinking water from public places and homes. Then she tests the water for microbes and harmful chemicals. If she finds anything harmful in the water, she tells the community's water department. The water department keeps people from drinking the water until the water is safe to drink.

Some health workers work with people. Mrs. Leech is a school nurse. She helps the students in her school. She tests their hearing and eyes. She keeps track of their height during the school year. And she takes care of students who become ill at school.

In what ways are a water inspector and a school nurse health workers?

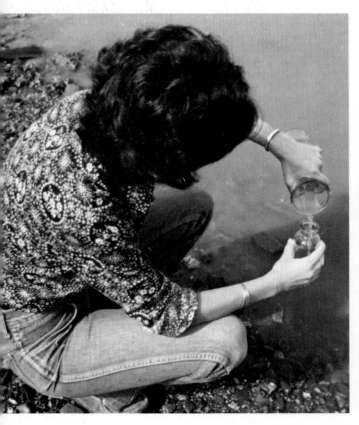

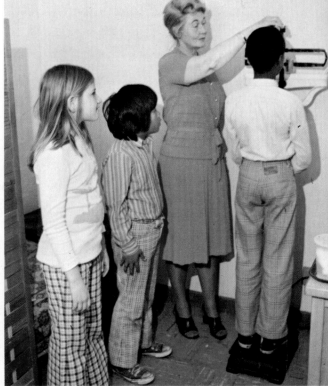

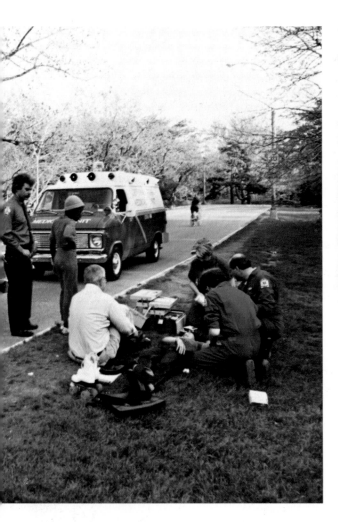

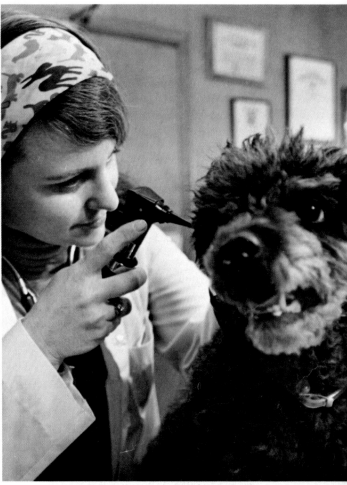

Other kinds of health workers also help when people become ill. Someone who is very ill may have to be taken to a hospital quickly in an ambulance. The ambulance has special equipment and trained workers. The ambulance workers take care of the person on the way to the hospital.

Some health workers take care of animals. Ms. Rosen is a veterinarian. She helps sick animals. She also gives animals vaccinations to keep them from getting certain diseases. Animals sometimes carry serious diseases that people can catch. By vaccinating animals, Ms. Rosen is helping to keep people healthy, too.

What kind of health workers are helping the person who is very sick? What kind of health worker is taking care of this dog?

About Veterinarians

Veterinarians also care for animals that give us foods. This helps make sure the food we eat is healthful.

Drawing a Fire-Safety Map

Draw a map of your neighborhood. On your map, label where all the fire alarm boxes are. If there is a fire station in your neighborhood, label it on your map, too.

What kind of community worker is a fire fighter?

Safety Workers

Other special helpers in your community work to keep people safe. These people are **safety workers.** They help keep accidents from happening. Sometimes they take care of people who have been in accidents.

Some safety workers help in an emergency. Mr. Antonini is a fire fighter. He helps in emergencies. He also works to keep emergencies from happening. Sometimes he explains fire safety rules to people. By following these rules, people can keep many fires from starting.

Mr. Antonini also tells people what to do if a fire starts. He explains where fire exits are located in a building. He also tells people in the building what to do if they cannot get out and have to wait to be rescued.

Sometimes Mr. Antonini helps in other emergencies, too. If someone were trapped in a car after an accident, Mr. Antonini could help rescue the person.

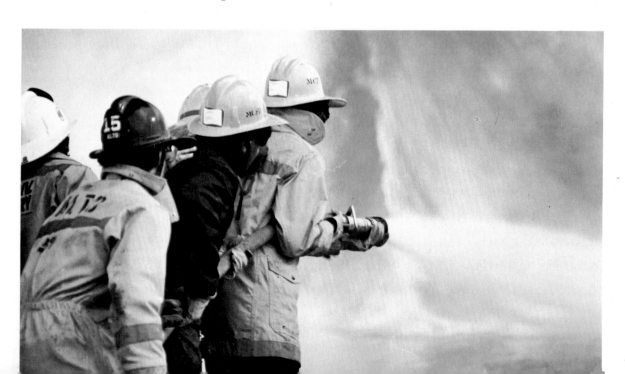

Ms. Asher is a police officer. She helps in emergencies. She works to keep accidents from happening, too. Officer Asher talks to young people. She shows them how to ride their bicycles safely. She tells people how to drive their cars safely. She also shows people ways to make their homes safe.

Every community has health and safety workers. They help keep you and everyone in your community healthy and safe.

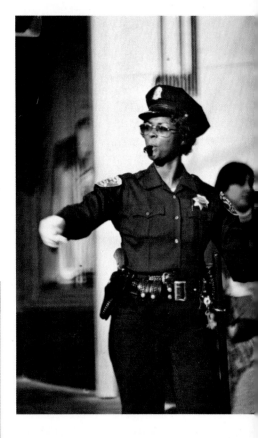

How might a police officer keep traffic accidents from happening?

Fire Safety Rules

- Keep lit matches and hot cigarette ashes away from materials that can burn.
- Make sure that a match is out and that its tip is cold before throwing it away.
- Keep matches away from young children.
- Keep furniture, clothing, rugs, and paper away from heaters.
- Store paint thinner in a metal or glass container with a tight lid. Keep it away from heat.
- Throw away oily rags. Do not let them pile up around the house.
- Make sure electrical wires are in good condition. Replace damaged wires at once.

REVIEW IT NOW

1. What is a community?
2. What is your environment?
3. What do health workers do?
4. How does a veterinarian help keep people healthy?
5. What do safety workers do?

Forestry Technician

Health Career

Many people enjoy hiking and camping in forests. But they may not know that forests are carefully tended and protected. The *forestry technician* cares for and protects forest lands.

Forestry technicians do many important jobs. They teach people about fire safety. They help put out fires, too. After a fire, forestry technicians inspect and report the damage. Then they help plant new trees.

Forestry technicians usually must have two years of college training. To learn more about being a forestry technician, write to the Society of American Foresters, 5400 Grosvenor Lane, Bethesda, MD 20814.

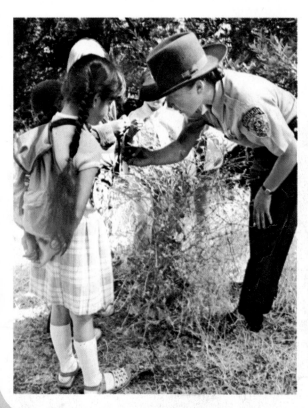
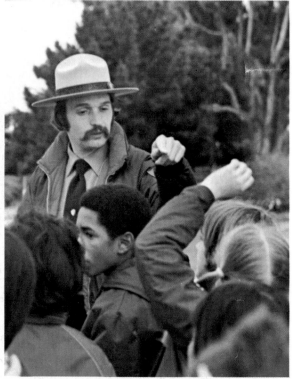

FOLLOWING COMMUNITY RULES

Communities have rules to protect all the people in the community. Community rules help people stay healthy and safe. You need to know and follow the health and safety rules of your community.

Why We Need Rules

Some rules protect people from accidents that could happen in unsafe places. The sign on the fence tells people to keep out of this vacant lot. Someone could be hurt playing here. Children playing on the blocks could fall.

Some rules protect people who must work in unsafe places. This is a "hard hat" area. The construction workers are putting up a new building. They are using heavy tools and materials that could fall and hit someone on the head. Wearing hard hats protects the workers' heads.

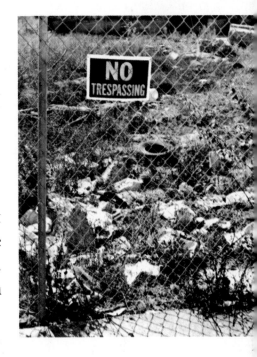

What is one reason to keep out of this vacant lot?

Why are these workers wearing hard hats?

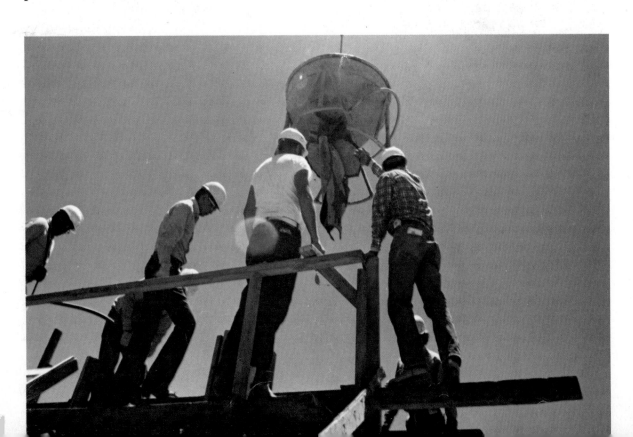

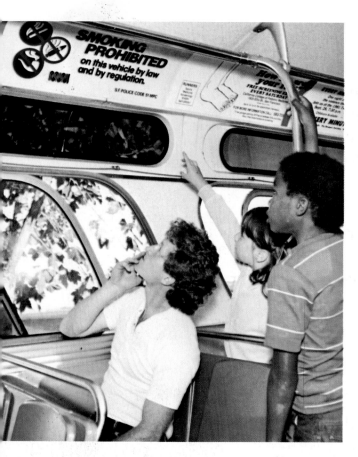

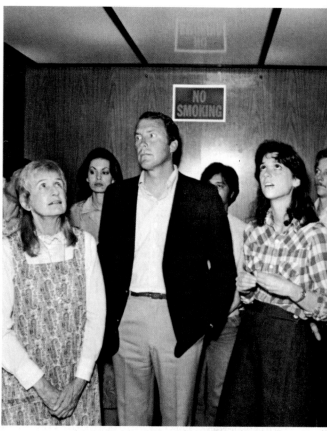

What is one reason for rules that prevent smoking in public places?

Some rules protect people's health. Tina and Ron are riding on the bus. A man near them is smoking. Tina points to the sign that forbids smoking and asks the man to put out his cigarette.

People who smoke in public places make other people breathe the smoke. The smoke is harmful to their health. Many communities have rules that forbid smoking in public places such as buses or elevators.

Other places have health and safety rules, too. Your school has many rules to protect you. You probably have health and safety rules at home, too. These rules are not written down. But everyone in the family knows them. These rules help keep you and your family safe and healthy.

Listing Home Health and Safety Rules

What health and safety rules do you have in your home? List at least three rules. How does each rule protect you or others?

Who Reminds Us to Follow Rules

Sometimes people in a community need to be reminded about the rules. Signs may remind them. Amy and Peter are riding their bicycles by the hospital. The hospital sign says, "Quiet, Hospital Zone." The sign reminds Amy and Peter that they should not make noise near the hospital.

Sometimes safety workers remind people to obey community rules. Officer Waldron is talking to Gerald and Sheila. He is reminding them that they should cross the street only with a green light or a WALK sign. They could be hurt if they crossed at any other time. A car could hit them. Or they could cause an accident in which other people are hurt.

Talking About Safety Signs

Signs in the community often remind people to follow health and safety rules. With a friend, talk about safety signs you have seen near your school. What might happen if someone did not obey the rules on the signs?

What are two ways people are reminded about community rules?

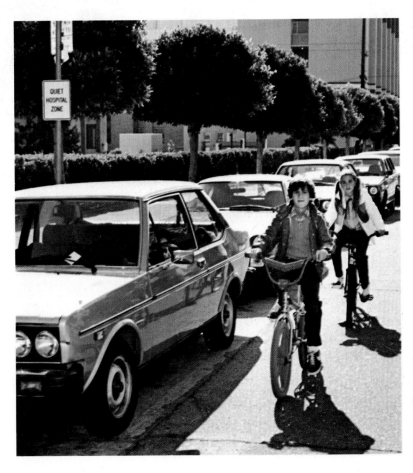

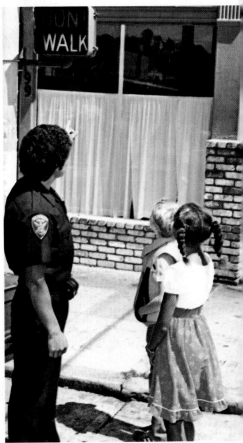

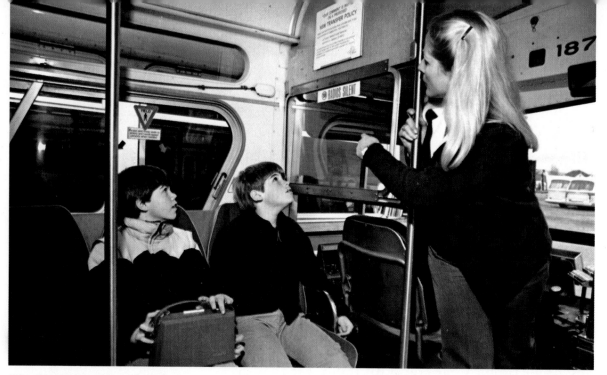

Why is there a rule to keep radios silent on public buses?

Doug and Ted are breaking a safety rule. The rule is on the sign above them. The sign says, "RADIOS SILENT." Doug and Ted have turned their radio on anyway. They are making the bus very noisy.

The bus driver reminds Doug and Ted about the rule. She asks them to turn off their radio. The driver tells the boys that loud noises from their radio could make her have an accident.

Sometimes you may forget a community rule. But your community has ways to remind you so that you can keep yourself and others healthy and safe.

REVIEW IT NOW

1. Why do communities need rules?
2. Why do communities have rules against smoking in public places?
3. What safety worker might remind you to obey a community rule?

GUARDING YOUR COMMUNITY AGAINST POLLUTION

Your community depends on its environment. Everyone in the community needs air and water. Everyone depends on the soil in which food grows. The community depends on plants and animals, too. If your environment is healthy, your community can stay healthy.

Changes in the Environment

People change their environment by using it. They take food, air, and water from the environment. They take trees for wood and paper. They take oil or coal for fuel. Sometimes they harm the environment. Other times they change the environment to make it better.

How can replanting trees taken for wood and paper help the environment?

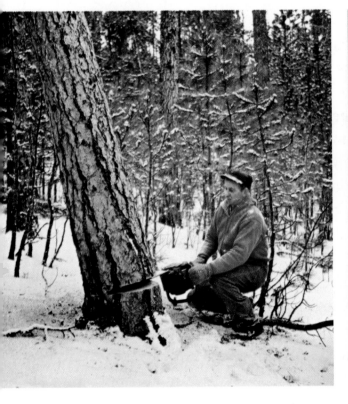

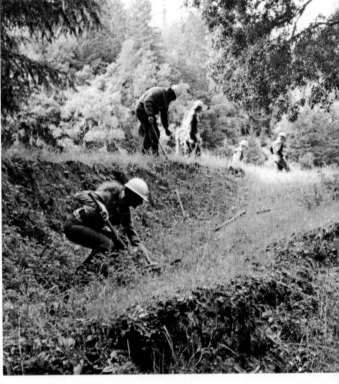

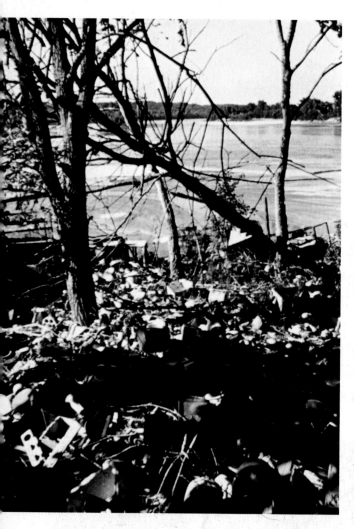

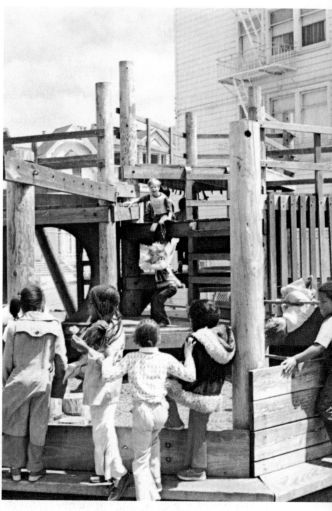

How can cleaning up a polluted environment help keep people healthy?

People can harm the environment by adding unhealthful matter to it. Unhealthful matter in the environment is **pollution.** People have harmed the shore of this lake. They have left litter on the beach. They have killed the water plants. They have **polluted,** or harmed, their environment and made it unhealthy.

People have changed this city environment for the better. They have picked up litter. They have built safe places for children to play. They have changed their neighborhood into a healthy environment.

Ed Pommerening

Ed Pommerening works in Idaho for a mining company. He replants trees on land that the mining company has used. But Ed has found an unusual way to do his job.

Ed noticed that only a few plants would grow in the used soil. So, he searched for a place with better growing conditions. Ed found the place—inside one of the mines! Now Ed has a plant nursery inside the mine. He tends the tiny seedlings there until they are strong. Then he plants them in the outside soil.

Ed has helped other companies grow their trees underground, too. Someday he even hopes to grow food crops underground.

Focus On

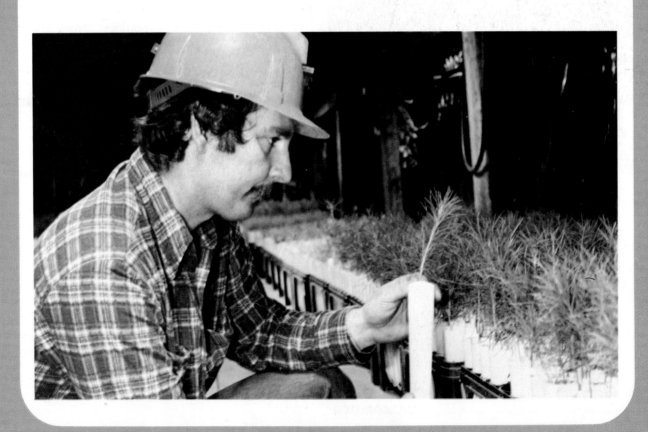

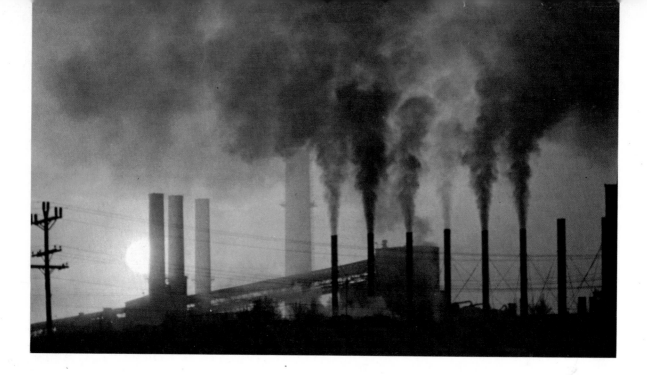

What are four ways air pollution can harm your health?

Air Pollution

Dirt and harmful matter in the air is **air pollution.** You can see smoke and dust that pollute the air. Some gases pollute the air, too, but you cannot see them.

Air pollution harms people's health in many ways. It can make people's eyes sting or "water." It can cause people to have trouble breathing. It can cause certain lung diseases or make other lung diseases worse.

Air pollution can harm trees and other plants. Plants give off oxygen. You need to breathe oxygen to stay alive. If there are fewer plants, the air has less oxygen. By killing plants, air pollution can harm people's health.

Some factories used to pollute the air but do not any more. Harmful matter is removed from these factories' wastes. The people who run these factories are taking better care of their community's environment.

About Air Pollution

In 1970, the **Clean Air Act** was passed to control sources of air pollution so that the air we breathe is not harmful to our health.

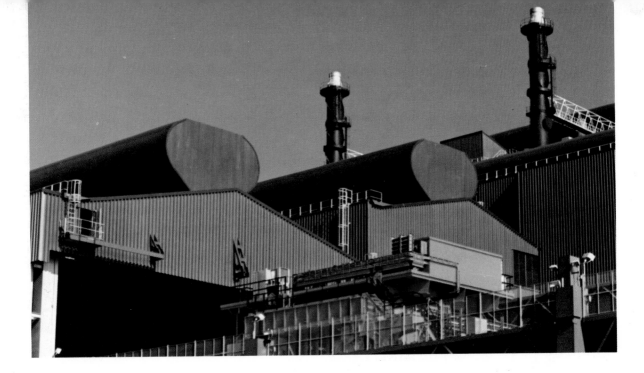

The companies that make cars, trucks, and buses are also working to cut down on air pollution. They are changing the engines so that the cars, trucks, and buses will put fewer harmful gases into the air.

How can removing harmful matter from a factory's wastes help the environment?

You can help stop air pollution, too. You can take a bus instead of asking to be driven somewhere in a car. One bus carrying 30 people causes less pollution than 30 cars carrying one person each. You can also walk or ride your bicycle instead of going in a car.

Smog Alert

Sometimes the smog in an area becomes so bad that it is dangerous to health. When this happens, city officials call a **smog alert.** The smog alert warns people of the unhealthful air. During a smog alert, people should not run or do other exercises outside. They should drive their cars only when necessary. They should stay inside as much as possible.

Water Pollution

Harmful matter in oceans, lakes, and rivers is called **water pollution.** Trash thrown into water causes water pollution. Chemicals from factories and oil from ships often pollute water. Wastes from people and animals can cause water pollution, too.

Polluted water often contains harmful microbes. Drinking or swimming in polluted water can make you ill. Water pollution also can kill plants and animals that live in and near water.

Many communities clean up water before using it. Most communities have water-treatment plants that remove microbes and wastes from water. Then the water is safe for people in the community to use.

Communities also can work to prevent water pollution. Many communities have treatment plants that treat wastes from people's houses. These plants remove solid materials from the water. They also kill most of the harmful microbes in the water. Then the treated water can be piped into lakes or rivers without causing pollution.

How do waste treatment plants help keep water safe for people to use?

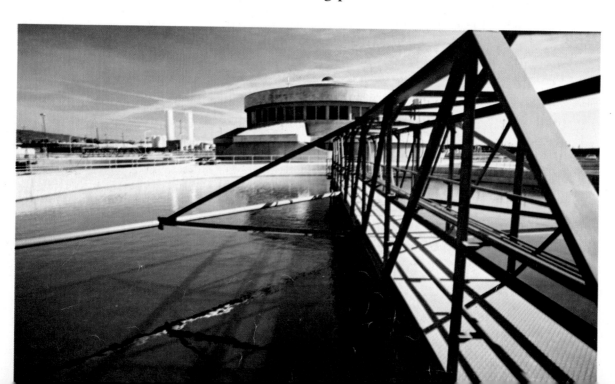

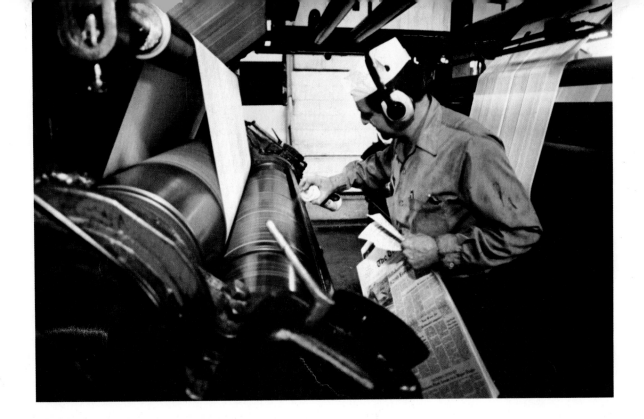

Noise Pollution

In what way is this worker avoiding harm from noise pollution?

Too much noise in the environment is **noise pollution.** It has many causes. Outside, noise pollution can be caused by car horns honking, loud sirens, or the roar of airplanes. In people's homes, noise pollution can be caused by television sets, radios, or record players turned up too loud. Noisy machinery in factories causes noise pollution, too.

Too much noise can harm people's health. It can make them nervous, cause them to have trouble sleeping, or make them get tired easily. Sudden noise can make a person's heart beat faster. A noisy place can cause people to lose their hearing for a while or even permanently.

People who run factories can prevent noise pollution in some ways. They can use machines that make less noise. They can provide special earmuffs or earplugs to protect the workers' hearing.

Loss of Hearing

Listening to loud music is one cause of hearing loss in teenagers. Stereo headphones may cause even more hearing loss. Many times people turn up the volume too loud. With headphones on, the loud music can cause damage to parts of the inner ear.

Talking About Noise Pollution

What are some causes of noise pollution in your community? What causes noise pollution in your school? Talk with classmates about what could be done to reduce noise pollution in your community and school.

Some communities try to cut down on noise by passing laws. Some laws keep car drivers from honking their horns except in an emergency. Other laws keep noisy factories from operating at night. Other laws keep airplanes from landing or taking off during certain hours of the day.

You can help prevent noise pollution. You can keep the volume on your television, radio, or record player turned down low. You should not play noisy games where you will bother other people. Doing these things will help make your environment less noisy.

Solid Waste Pollution

Trash, garbage, and litter are called **solid wastes.** When they pile up in open dumps or pollute the environment, they cause **solid waste pollution.** This kind of pollution makes the environment unhealthful and ugly. Harmful microbes can grow in

How can solid waste pollution harm your health?

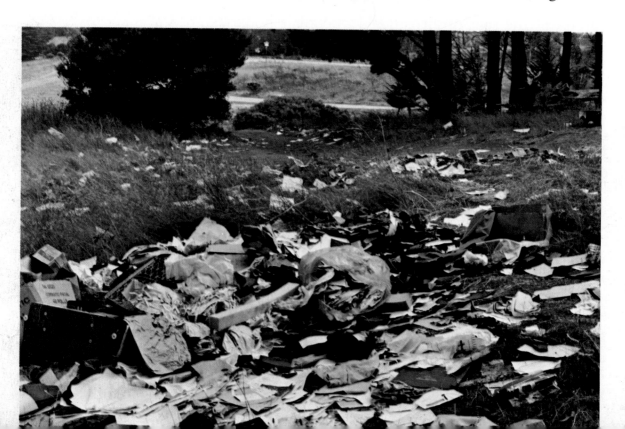

garbage dumped in the open. Rats and insects eat the garbage. They can spread the microbes to people and may cause illness.

Communities must get rid of their solid wastes in ways that do not pollute the environment. Trash can be burned, but that causes air pollution. When trash is dumped into rivers or lakes, it causes water pollution. Most communities have found better ways than these to prevent solid waste pollution.

Landfills

Some communities bury their trash. First, workers pick up the trash from people's houses. Then they take the trash to a special dumping place. There, other workers bury the trash. Land with trash buried in it is called a **landfill.**

After the landfill is full of buried trash, the land can be used in different ways. The land can be used as a park. Or the land can be used for building houses or offices.

What might some communities do after a landfill is filled with trash?

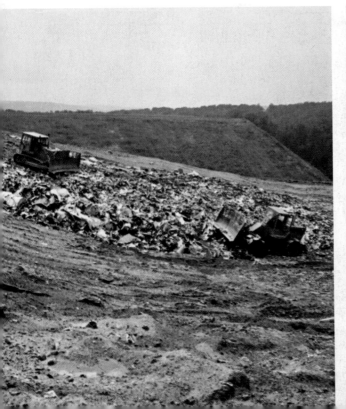

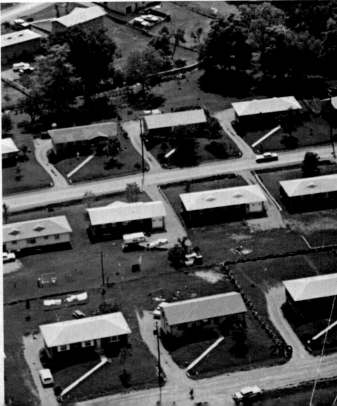

The Baltimore Heat Plant

Baltimore, Maryland, has found a way to get rid of solid wastes and produce energy, too.

Each day, tons of garbage are shredded to small bits and burned in a hot furnace. The furnace is so hot that the wastes are broken down into gases and ash. Then the gases are burned to make steam. A local power plant uses the steam to heat and air condition office buildings. One source says the Baltimore Heat Plant makes twice as much energy as it uses!

Baltimore plans to open a second garbage-energy plant. The new plant will be able to change twice as much garbage into energy.

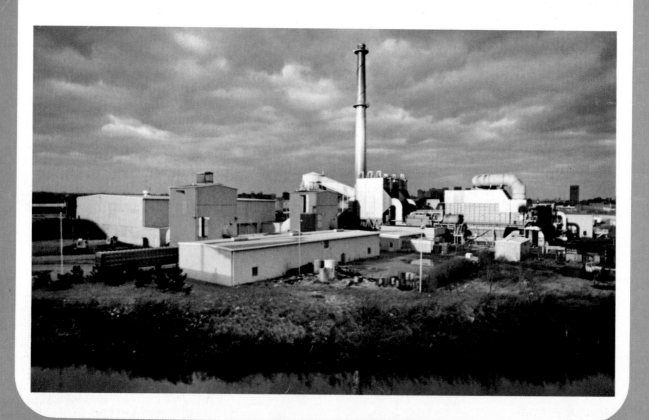

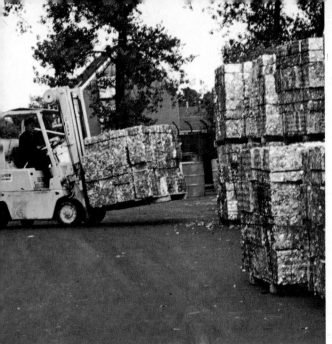
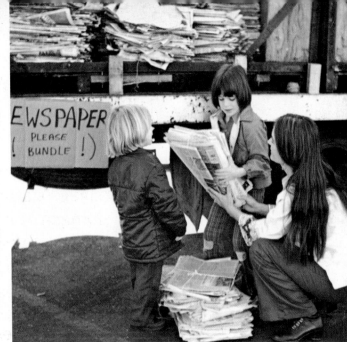

Recycling

Other communities prevent solid waste pollution by making their trash useful again. They reuse, or **recycle,** many kinds of trash.

This city picks metal out of its trash. The metal will be melted down and used to make new cans. The metal will not pollute the city or be wasted, either.

Paper can be recycled, too. Old newspapers can be shredded and made into new paper. Recycling paper cuts down on solid waste pollution. It also helps the environment in another way. It saves trees. Paper is made from trees. When people recycle paper, they use up fewer trees.

Glass bottles and jars can also be recycled. The glass is broken up and melted down. Then it is made into new glass.

Many communities have special places called **recycling centers.** People bring their old cans, bottles, and newspapers to the centers to be recycled. Then the trash does not pollute the community's environment.

How can recycling metal, paper, and glass prevent solid waste pollution?

Finding Out About Recycling Centers

Look in your telephone book and find out if your community has any recycling centers. If it does, where are they? When is each one open? What materials are recycled at each center? How do you have to prepare each material for the center?

241

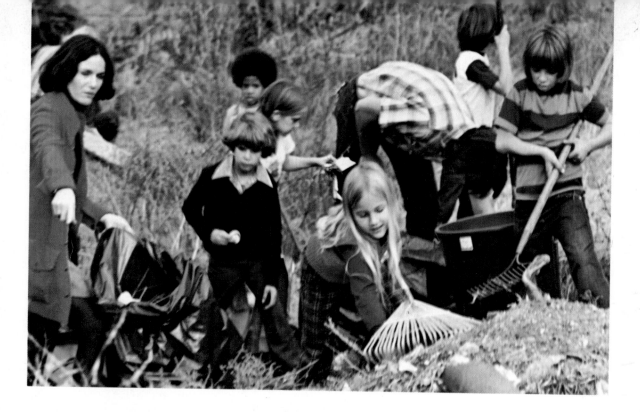

How are these children helping to keep their environment healthy?

You can help prevent solid waste pollution. You can put trash into a trash can instead of littering. If you see litter, you can pick it up. You can also take cans, bottles, and paper to a recycling center.

Almost everything people do changes the environment in some way. Some of these changes harm the environment by causing pollution. You can help keep your community and your environment healthy by trying to prevent pollution.

REVIEW IT NOW

1. What is pollution?
2. What are three causes of air pollution?
3. What is one way you can prevent air pollution?
4. What is water pollution?
5. How can noise pollution harm people's health?
6. What are two ways communities can prevent solid waste pollution?

Making a Pollution Prevention Chart

You and your family can help your community prevent pollution. Make a "Pollution Prevention" chart to show how you can help.

Use a piece of poster paper for your chart. Make four columns on the paper. Write "Air," "Water," "Noise," and "Solid Waste" at the top of each column. Discuss with your family how you can prevent each kind of pollution. Then write down what you can do. You may want to draw or use pictures to show what you can do, too.

Keep your chart where you and your family can see it. Use it as a reminder to help you keep your community free of pollution.

Working Toward Wellness

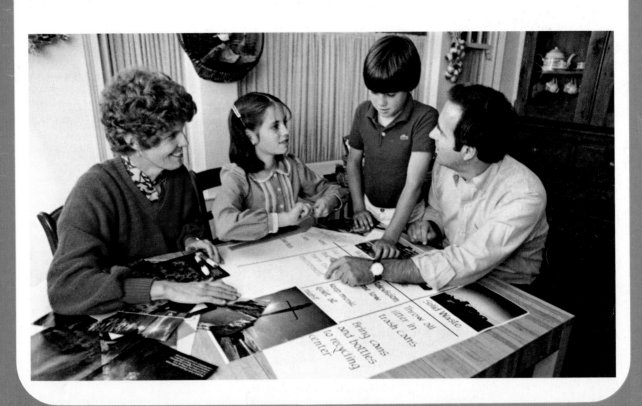

To Help You Review

Checking Your Understanding

Write the numbers from 1 to 12 on your paper. After each number, write the answer to the question or questions. Page numbers in ( ) tell you where to look in the chapter if you need help.

1. In what way is a family like a community? (**220**)
2. What are six different things the environment includes? (**220**)
3. What are five different kinds of health workers? (**221–223**)
4. What kinds of safety workers might help keep accidents from happening? How? (**224–225**)
5. Why might construction workers have to wear hard hats? (**227**)
6. What are three ways air pollution may harm a person's health? (**234**)
7. What are three causes of water pollution? (**236**)
8. In what way does a water treatment plant make water safe to use? (**236**)
9. How do some communities try to cut down on noise pollution? (**238**)
10. Why have many communities found better ways than burning and dumping to get rid of trash? (**239**)
11. What is a landfill? (**239**)
12. What are three kinds of materials that can be recycled? (**241**)

Checking Your Health Vocabulary

Write the numbers from 1 to 8 on your paper. After each number, write the letter of the meaning for the word or words. Page numbers in ( ) tell you where to look in the chapter if you need help.

1. community (**220**)
2. environment (**220**)
3. health workers (**221**)
4. safety workers (**224**)
5. pollution (**232**)
6. solid wastes (**238**)
7. recycle (**241**)
8. recycling centers (**241**)

a. trash, garbage, and litter
b. community workers who help keep people safe
c. to reuse, or make useful again
d. everything in and around a community
e. a group of people who depend on one another
f. unhealthful matter in the environment
g. community workers who help prevent disease
h. places where people bring old cans, bottles, and newspapers to be used again

Write the numbers from 9 to 12 on your paper. Then write a sentence that explains each kind of pollution. Page numbers in ( ) tell you where to look in the chapter if you need help.

9. air pollution (**234**)
10. water pollution (**236**)
11. noise pollution (**237**)
12. solid waste pollution (**238**)

Practice Test

True or False?

Write the numbers from 1 to 10 on your paper. After each number, write *T* if the sentence is *true*. Write *F* if it is *false*. Rewrite each false sentence to make it true.

1. All the people in a community depend on the same environment.
2. A community's environment includes only nonliving things, such as air, water, and soil.
3. A veterinarian takes care of sick children.
4. Some safety workers take care of people who have been hurt in accidents.
5. Sometimes signs remind people to follow health and safety rules.
6. People change the environment by using it.
7. Air pollution can harm people but not plants.
8. Polluted water can harm only people who drink it.
9. Some ways of getting rid of solid waste materials pollute the environment.
10. Recycling paper can help save trees.

Complete the Sentence

Write the numbers from 11 to 20 on your paper. After each number, copy the sentence and fill in the missing word.

11. Food inspectors and water inspectors are two kinds of _____ workers.
12. An _____ has special equipment and can take someone to a hospital very quickly.
13. Most communities have health and safety _____ for people to follow.
14. A rule that forbids smoking in a public place is an example of a _____ rule.
15. Smoke from factories may cause _____ pollution.
16. Polluted water may contain harmful _____.
17. Loud machinery, sirens, and honking car horns are sources of _____ pollution.
18. Some communities bury _____ in landfills and use the land again.
19. _____ can be melted down and used again to make new cans.
20. People bring old cans, bottles, and newspapers to _____ centers.

Learning More

For You to Do

1. Make a list of at least ten things in your community's environment. Include nonliving things such as buildings and cars. Include living things such as people and animals. Put an **O** by each thing that makes you healthy. Put an **X** by each thing that harms your health. Then look at your list. How can you help improve your environment?

2. Imagine you are in a noisy place. You might be in a school lunch room, at home, or on a bus. You might be trying to write, think, or read. With a group of your classmates, act out a situation like this. Show your feelings about being in a noisy place. Show what you can do to try to make the place less noisy.

For You to Find Out

1. Find out what different things a health worker, such as your school nurse, does each day. How does each of these activities protect your community's health?

2. What is *thermal pollution?* What causes it? Does thermal pollution happen as often as air pollution? How can thermal pollution harm living things in rivers or lakes? Use library books to help you find out about this kind of pollution.

3. Certain stores take in clothing or household goods that people no longer want. Often, they fix them and then sell them for a low price. Find out whether your community has stores like this. You might look in the Yellow Pages of a telephone book for used clothing or household goods. How are these stores like recycling centers?

For You to Read

Here are some books you can look for in your school or public library to find out more about your environment.

Santrey, Laurence. *Conservation and Pollution*. Troll Associates, 1985.

Woods, Geraldine, and Woods, Harold. *Pollution*. Franklin Watts, 1985.

EXERCISE HANDBOOK

This special part of your health book is about exercise. It shows you exercises that are fun and easy to do. These exercises can help you feel good and look good. They can help you lose weight. They can help your heart and lungs work well. And they can help you relax.

The Exercise Handbook is divided into four parts: "Stretching Out," "Individual Exercise," "Group Exercise," and "Cooling Down."

You should exercise at least every other day for 15 minutes or more. Exercising in this way can help you reach wellness. Exercising will help you now and throughout your life. Before you begin your exercise program, be sure to check with your doctor. Some exercises may not be safe for you. Your doctor is the only person who can decide which exercises you should do and which ones you should not do.

STRETCHING OUT

Every time you exercise, begin by stretching out the muscles of your body. Stretching out your muscles helps prevent them from being injured when you exercise hard. Here are some stretching exercises you can do before playing a game or sport. Each of these exercises stretches a different group of muscles. You should do several exercises each time you stretch out in order to stretch different groups of muscles.

Side Bends

1. Stand with your feet about as far apart as the width of your shoulders. Put your left hand on your waist and raise your right hand above your head.

2. Bend your body to the left as shown in picture 1. Bend until you feel a "pull" at your waist. Hold that position for 5 seconds.

3. Repeat step 2 five times.

4. Raise your other arm above your head.

5. Repeat steps 2 and 3 to the right side.

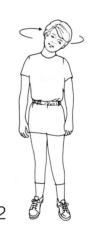

1

Head Rolls

1. Stand with your legs slightly apart and your arms at your sides.

2. Gently roll your head in a circle as shown in picture 2. As your roll it forward, try to touch your chest with your chin.

3. Repeat step 2, but roll your head in the opposite direction.

4. Repeat steps 2 and 3 in order four times.

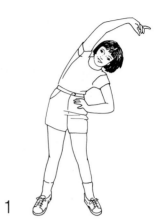

2

Lying-Down Knee Lifts

1. Lie on your back with your legs stretched out and close together.

2. Keeping your back on the floor, raise your right knee. Grasp it with both hands, and pull it gently toward your chest as shown in picture 3. Hold this position for 5 seconds.

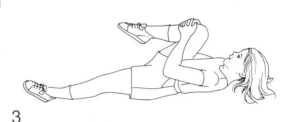

3

3. Return to the position in step 1.

4. Repeat steps 2 and 3 using your left knee.

5. Repeat steps 2 through 4 five times.

Slow Jog

1. Stand with your feet a few inches apart and your elbows slightly bent.

2. Slowly jog in place as shown in picture 4. Jog for about 30 seconds.

3. When you have finished jogging take two deep breaths.

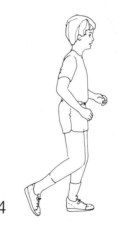

4

INDIVIDUAL EXERCISE

Here is an exercise you can do by yourself that can help your heart and lungs stay healthy. Before starting this exercise, do some stretching movements. Then do the exercise hard enough to speed up your pulse and breathing. Keep exercising for at least twelve minutes after your pulse and breathing have speeded up. You can do more than one exercise as long as you do not stop to rest between exercises.

Jumping Jacks

1. Stand with your feet together and your arms at your sides.

2. Jump up, spread your feet apart and swing your arms up. Land in the position shown in picture 5. Your feet should be a little further apart that the width of your shoulders.

3. Jump up again. As you jump, bring your feet together and your arms down. Land in the starting position.

4. Repeat steps 2 and 3 in an even rhythm ten times.

5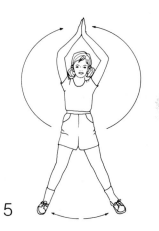

GROUP EXERCISE

Playing an active game with your friends is a good way to exercise and have fun at the same time. Here is an active game that you and your friends might have fun playing. Remember to stretch out well before you start playing any active game.

Pass and Catch

Here is a game you can play with 10 or more people. You will need a playing field or area with a goal line on each side. The lines should be between 25 and 60 feet (7.5 m and 18.2 m) apart. You will also need a football.

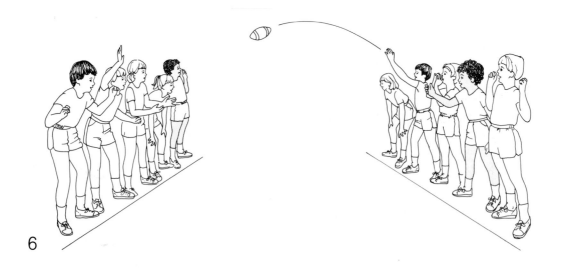

6

1. Divide the players into two teams. Each team should stand behind its own goal line as shown in picture 6. Teams should be facing each other.

2. To begin the game, a player on one team throws the ball over the line of the other players.

3. All the players on the other team stand on the goal line when the ball is thrown. Then any player can run and catch the ball.

4. If no player on the other team catches the ball, or if the ball touches the ground before a player catches it, the team that threw the ball gets a point.

5. If a player on the other team catches the ball before it touches the ground, no point is scored.

6. If the ball does *not* go over the goal line, any player on the other team may run forward to catch it. If the player catches the ball in front of the goal line, his or her team gets a point.

7. Teams should take turns throwing the ball. Every player on each team should have a chance to throw the ball before the game is ended.

8. The team that has the most points wins the game.

COOLING DOWN

Always end your exercising with a few exercises that will allow your body to cool down slowly. You can use many of the same exercises for cooling down as for stretching out. For cooling down, however, you should do an exercise fewer times than for stretching out. You should also do the exercise more slowly. Here are some exercises you can use to cool down

Body Twists

1. Lie on your back with your legs straight. Stretch your arms out from your shoulders.

2. Lift your right leg straight up. Cross it over your left leg as shown in picture 7.

3. Bring your leg back to the straight-up position.

4. Lower your leg to its position in step 1.

5. Repeat steps 2 through 4 with your left leg.

6. Complete steps 2 through 5 three times.

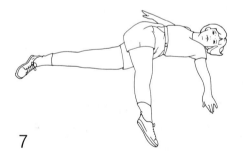
7

Forward and Backward Bends

1. Stand with your back to a wall and your arms at your sides. You should be about one foot (30 cm) from the wall. Breathe deeply.

2. Let your air out slowly while bending your knees and the rest of your body. You should end up in the position shown in picture 8.

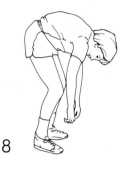

8

3. When you have let out all your breath, begin taking air in again slowly. As you breathe in, raise your body slowly back to the position in step 1.

4. Raise your arms above your head. Bend backward until your fingertips touch the wall as shown in picture 9. Then return to the position in step 1.

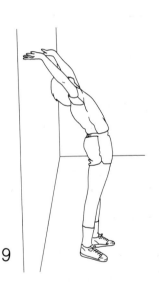

9

5. Complete steps 2 through 4 three times.

6. Finish by taking two deep breaths. Then relax and let your body rest.

GLOSSARY

This glossary contains major health words and their definitions introduced in this text. A page number follows each definition. It tells where to find the word in the text.

Each glossary word is in **dark** type. The correct pronunciation of each word is given in the special spelling in ( ) after that word. For example, the word <u>accident</u> appears this way: **ac·ci·dent** ('ak-səd-ənt).

The sounds used in the spellings in ( ) are explained in the Pronunciation Key below. Each symbol or letter stands for a sound. You can recognize this sound in the words following it.

Most glossary words have the mark ' placed before a syllable. This mark shows you that the syllable is pronounced with more force, or stress, than the other syllables in the word, as in the entry **al·co·hol** ('al-kə-hȯl).

Pronunciation Key

a	cat, lap, bad	j	jet, germ, just	<u>th</u>	that, there
ā	say, late, take	k	keep, crawl	ü	rude, booth
ä	father, lot	l	pale	u̇	put, stood
au̇	cow, shout, mouth	m	man, him	v	river
b	bubble, bib	n	not, loan	w	wall, power
ch	chill	ŋ	linger, young	y	you, yellow
d	dot, do	ō	tone, hope	yü	fuel, mule
e	let, red	ȯ	law, tall	yu̇	pure
ē	meat, cheese	ȯi	join	z	gaze, rise
f	puff	p	cap	zh	decision
g	got, bag	r	bread, far	ə	(represents)
h	happy	s	soul, moss		a in amount
hw	white, where	sh	shut, ocean		e in thicken
i	lip, give	t	tap		i in edible
ī	bite, tie	th	tooth, within		o in cannon
					u in catsup

A

ac·ci·dent ('ak-səd-ənt), unexpected event that can harm a person's health. **190**

ac·ids ('as-ədz), sour substances that can break down tooth enamel. **94**

air pol·lu·tion (aər pə-'lü-shən), dirt and harmful matter in the air. **234**

air sacs (saks), tiny, balloonlike sacs in the lungs. **42**

al·co·hol ('al-kə-hȯl), drug found in drinks like beer, wine, and whiskey. **170**

al·co·hol·ics (al-kə-'hȯl-iks), people who have a disease called alcoholism. **180**

al·co·hol·ism ('al-kə-hȯ-liz-əm), disease in which people need alcohol to feel normal and become ill when they try to stop drinking. **180**

an·ti·body ('ant-i-bäd-ē), substance made by white blood cells to stop certain disease microbes from acting. **150**

ar·ter·ies ('ärt-ə-rez), blood vessels that carry blood away from the heart. **46**

B

bac·te·ria (bak-'tir-ē-ə), one group of microbes that can cause disease. **136**

bal·anced di·et ('bal-ənst 'di-ət), diet that includes food from each of the four basic food groups. **75**

ball-and-sock·et joint (bȯl-ənd-'säk-ət jȯint), kind of joint that lets one bone move in a circle. **34**

bi·cus·pids (bi-'kəs-pədz), back teeth with two points for grinding and crushing food. **89**

blood (bləd), liquid that carries food and oxygen to the cells. **44**

blood ves·sels ('ves-əlz), small tubes that carry blood to and from all parts of the body. **44**

body sys·tem ('bäd-ē 'sis-təm), organs working together on the same job. **30**

boost·er ('bü-stər), vaccine given again when immunity to a disease only lasts a short time. **153**

brain (brān), organ that is used to think and that tells every other part of the body what to do. **49**

C

caf·feine (ka-'fēn), drug found in coffee, tea, and cola drinks that speeds up the heart, the nerves, and many other parts of the body. **169**

cal·cu·lus ('kal-kyə-ləs), hard, yellow substance that forms from plaque that has stayed on the teeth too long. **95**

cap·il·lar·ies ('kap-ə-ler-ēz), tiny blood vessels that connect arteries to veins. **46**

car·bon di·ox·ide ('kar-bən dī-'äk-sīd), gas the cells make but cannot use. **41**

car·bon mon·ox·ide (mə-'näk-sīd), gas in tobacco smoke that takes the place of oxygen in a smoker's blood. **172**

cav·i·ty ('kav-ət-ē), hole in a tooth. **94**

cells, smallest living parts of the body. **28**

cir·cu·la·to·ry sys·tem ('sər-kyə-lə-tōr-ē 'sis-təm), body system that carries food materials and oxygen to all the cells and carries away wastes. **44**

com·mu·ni·ca·ble dis·eases (kə-'myü-ni-kə-bəl diz-'ēz-əz), diseases that pass from one person to another. **135**

com·mu·ni·ty (kə-'myü-nət-ē), group of people who depend on one another. **220**

crown, part of a tooth a person can see. **92**

cus·pids ('kəs-pədz), teeth on either side of the incisors that tear food. **88**

D

de·cay (di-'kā), to rot. **94**

de·fenses (di-'fens-əz), ways the body has to fight against microbes. **149**

den·tal floss ('dent-əl fläs), special kind of white string that can remove plaque and food from between the teeth and clean along the gumline. **96**

den·tal hy·gien·ist (hī-'jēn-əst), person who cleans teeth and shows people how to care for their teeth. **96**

den·tin ('dent-ən), thick layer under the enamel of a tooth. **92**

di·et ('dī-ət), food a person eats daily. **75**

di·ges·tion (dī-'jes-chən), breaking up and changing of food. **38**

di·ges·tive juices (dī-'jes-tiv 'jüs-əz), special liquids that help digest food. **38**

di·ges·tive sys·tem (dī-'jes-tiv 'sis-təm), body system that breaks up food. **38**

dis·ease (diz-'ēz), any breakdown in the way the body works. **134**

dis·ease mi·crobes (diz-'ēz 'mī-krōbz), microbes that can cause disease when they enter the body. **138**

drug, any substance other than food that causes changes in the body. **162**

E

emer·gen·cy (i-'mər-jən-sē), serious accident for which help is needed right away. **193**

emo·tion·al needs (i-'mō-shnəl nēdz), needs that have to do with feelings. **12**

em·phy·se·ma (em-fə-'zē-mə), disease caused when tobacco smoke tears air sacs in the lungs. **173**

enam·el (in-'am-əl), thin, hard, outer layer of a tooth. **92**

en·vi·ron·ment (in-'vī-rən-mənt), everything in and around a community. **220**

esoph·a·gus (i-'säf-ə-gəs), tube made of muscle that squeezes food down into the stomach. **38**

ex·er·cise ('ek-sər-sīz), any activity that makes the body work hard. **108**

F

food group, group of foods that have almost the same nutrients. **74**

fun·gi ('fən-jī), one group of microbes that cannot move by themselves and that can cause disease. **137**

G

gums, pink tissue around the teeth. **92**

H

health work·ers, community workers who help prevent disease. **221**

heart, organ that pumps blood and keeps it moving through the body all the time. **44**

heart·beat ('härt-bēt), squeezing of blood into the blood vessels. **46**

hinge joint (hinj jöint), kind of joint that swings open and shut like a door on a hinge. **34**

I

im·mov·able joints (im-'mü-və-bəl jöints), joints that do not let the body move. **34**

im·mune (im-'yün), protected from a certain disease. **151**

im·mu·ni·ty (im-'yü-nət-ē), body's ability to defend itself with antibodies against microbes of a certain kind. **151**

in·ci·sors (in-'sī-zərz), front teeth with sharp edges and flat tops for cutting food. **88**

in·fec·tion (in-'fek-shən), growth of disease microbes somewhere inside the body. **139**

in·ner ear, part of the ear inside the head with which a person hears. **55**

J

joints (jöints), places in the body where bones connect. **34**

L

land·fill, land with trash buried in it. **239**

large in·tes·tine (lärj in-'tes-tən), organ that stores wastes from food. **40**

lung can·cer (ləng 'kan-sər), disease in which lumps grow inside the lungs. **173**

lungs (ləngz), large organs inside the chest for breathing. **42**

M

med·i·cines ('med-ə-sənz), drugs used to help fight illness. **163**

mi·crobes ('mī-krōbz), tiny living creatures that can make a person ill if enough of them get inside the body. **44**

mi·cro·scope ('mī-krə-skōp), viewing instrument that makes small things look bigger. **28**

mo·lars ('mō-lərz), wide teeth in the very back of the mouth for grinding and crushing food. **89**

mus·cles ('məs-əlz), organs of the muscular system. **36**

mus·cu·lar sys·tem ('məs-kyə-lər 'sis-təm), body system that helps the body move. **32**

N

needs, things a person must meet or satisfy to be healthy. **11**

nerve cells ('nərv selz), special cells that make up the nervous system. **49**

nerves (nərvz), bundles of long nerve cells. **50**

ner·vous sys·tem ('nər-vəs 'sis-təm), body system that controls the many things a person does. **49**

nic·o·tine ('nik-ə-tēn), drug in tobacco smoke that makes the openings of the blood vessels smaller than they should be. **172**

noise pol·lu·tion (nȯiz pə-'lü-shən), too much noise in the environment. **237**

non·com·mu·ni·ca·ble dis·eases (nön-kə-'myü-ni-kə-bəl diz-'ēz-əz), diseases that are not passed from one person to another. **135**

nu·tri·ents ('nü-trē-ənts), parts of food that help the body grow and give it energy. **70**

O

odors ('ōd-ərz), smells. **56**

or·gans ('ȯr-gənz), groups of tissues working together. **30**

out·er ear, part of the ear that people can see. **55**

over-the-coun·ter med·i·cines ('ō-vər-thə-'kaȯnt-ər 'med-ə-sənz), medicines that can be bought without a prescription; also called **OTC medicines. 167**

ox·y·gen ('äk-si-jən), gas that the cells need and that is in the air a person breathes. **41**

P

pe·des·tri·an (pə-'des-trē-ən), person who is walking. **199**

per·ma·nent teeth ('pərm-ə-nənt tēth), second set of teeth. **87**

per·son·al·i·ty (pərs-ən-'al-ət-ē), all the ways a person looks, thinks, feels, and acts. **9**

phar·ma·cist ('fär-mə-səst), specially trained worker who prepares medicines. **166**

phys·i·cal needs ('fiz-i-kəl nēdz), things the body needs to stay alive. **11**

phys·i·cal traits ('fiz-i-kəl trāts), traits that tell about the body. **6**

plaque (plak), clear, gooey substance that forms on teeth and is made up of food and microbes that stick together. **94**

plate·lets ('plāt-ləts), blood cells that help form a scab over a cut. **44**

pol·lute (pə-'lüt), to harm the environment by adding unhealthful matter to it. **232**

pol·lu·tion (pə-'lü-shən), unhealthful matter in the environment. **232**

pores (pōrz), small openings in the skin through which sweat leaves the body. **57**

pos·ture ('päs-chər), way a person holds his or her body. **112**

pre·scrip·tion (pri-'skrip-shən), order from a doctor for a medicine. **166**

pre·scrip·tion med·i·cines (pri-'skrip-shən 'med-ə-sənz), medicines that can be bought only with a prescription from a doctor. **166**

pri·ma·ry teeth ('prī-mer-ē tēth), first set of teeth. **87**

pro·to·zoa (prōt-ə-'zō-ə), one group of microbes that are the largest in size and that can move about on their own. **137**

pulp (pəlp), soft tissue with nerves and blood vessels inside a tooth. **92**

pulse (pəls), push of blood through the arteries with each heartbeat. **117**

R

re·cy·cle (rē-'sī-kəl), to reuse or make useful again. **241**

re·cy·cling cen·ters (rē-'sī-kliŋ 'sen-tərz), places where people bring old bottles, cans, and newspapers to be made useful again. **241**

red blood cells, tiny, round blood cells that carry oxygen to all the body's cells. **44**

re·sis·tance (ri-'zis-tənts), body's ability to fight off disease microbes. **153**

re·spi·ra·to·ry sys·tem ('res-pə-rə-tò-rē 'sis-təm), body system that helps a person breathe. **41**

root, hidden part of a tooth that goes through the gum and into the jawbone. **92**

S

safe·ty work·ers, community workers who help keep people safe. **224**

scab, blood that has dried on a cut forming a hard covering. **149**

sense (sens), to become aware of certain information about the world. **52**

senses ('sen-səz), seeing, hearing, smelling, tasting, and touching. **52**

side ef·fects (sīd i-'fekts), unneeded changes in the body caused by medicines. **164**

skel·e·tal sys·tem ('skel-ət-əl 'sis-təm), body system that gives the body its basic shape. **32**

skel·e·ton ('skel-ət-ən), all of the bones in the body. **32**

skull (skəl), rounded set of bones that covers the brain. **34**

small in·tes·tine (smól in-'tes-tən), organ where most digestion takes place. **40**

smog a·lert (smäg ə-'lərt), warning to people about unhealthful air. **235**

smoke·less to·bac·co (smōk-lis tə-'bak-ō), tobacco made to be put into the mouth and left there for a while. **170**

sol·id waste pol·lu·tion ('säl-əd wäst pə-'lü-shən), pollution caused by trash, garbage, and litter piled up in open dumps or in the environment. **238**

sol·id wastes, trash, garbage, and litter. **238**

spi·nal cord ('spīn-əl kòrd), large bundle of nerves down the back and connected to the brain. **50**

spine (spīn), stack of bones that protects the spinal cord. **50**

stom·ach ('stəm-ək), organ made of muscle that squeezes and mashes up food. **40**

sweat (swet), liquid waste from the skin. **57**

sweat glands, small organs in the skin that produce sweat. **57**

symp·toms ('simp-təmz), pains and other signs of disease. **134**

T

tar, sticky brown substance in tobacco smoke that coats the inside of the windpipe. **172**

taste buds, nerve cells inside bumps on the tongue that identify tastes. **56**

tis·sues ('tish-yüz), groups of the same kinds of cells working together. **29**

to·bac·co (tə-'bak-ō), filling inside cigarettes and cigars. **170**

trait (trāt), feature that tells something about a person. **4**

V

vac·ci·nat·ed ('vak-sə-nāt-əd), given a vaccine. **153**

vac·cines (vak-'sēnz), medicines that help the body form immunity to some diseases. **153**

veins (vānz), blood vessels that carry blood back to the heart. **46**

vi·ruses ('vī-rəs-əz), one group of microbes that are the smallest in size and that do not grow by dividing. **137**

W

wastes, materials that the body cannot use and must be removed from the body. **40**

wa·ter pol·lu·tion ('wȯt-ər pə-lü-shən), harmful matter in oceans, lakes, and rivers. **236**

wellness, highest level of health you can possibly reach. **5**

white blood cells, blood cells that help fight certain kinds of illness by attacking microbes. **44**

wind·pipe, tube for breathing that goes from the nose and mouth down into the chest. **42**

wis·dom teeth ('wiz-dəm tēth), four molars at the very back of the mouth. **90**

INDEX

D 9
E 0
F 1
G 2
H 3
I 4
J 5